# Nutraceuticals

# Nutraceuticals

Lisa Rapport

BPharm, MPhil, MRPharmS

Community Pharmacist and Researcher
School of Pharmacy and Pharmaceutical Sciences
University of Manchester, UK

Brian Lockwood

BPharm, PhD, MRPharmS

Lecturer
School of Pharmacy and Pharmaceutical Sciences
University of Manchester, UK

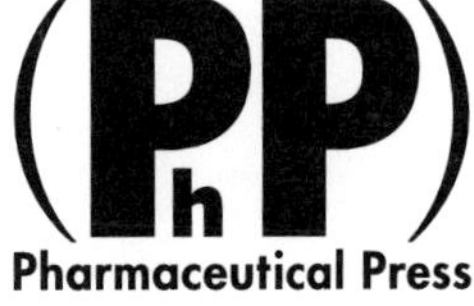

Published by the Pharmaceutical Press
1 Lambeth High Street, London SE1 7JN, UK

First published 2002



Text design by Barker/Hilsdon, Lyme Regis, Dorset
Typeset by Type Study, Scarborough, North Yorkshire
Printed in Great Britain by TJ International, Padstow, Cornwall

ISBN 0 85369 503 2



A catalogue record for this book is available from the British Library

# Contents

# Preface

We first thought up the idea of a book on nutraceuticals in the summer of 1997, when we realised that there was a gap in informed books on the subject of complementary medicines of natural origin that were not herbal remedies. At this time nutraceuticals were increasingly becoming available in the high street and by mail order. In fact any newspaper colour supplement would contain some advertisement for nutraceuticals, and complementary medicine articles in the lay press were increasingly promoting their virtues.

Just as with herbal remedies, many suppliers advertise a range of products as being of natural origin and thus presumably devoid of the problems associated with conventional pharmaceuticals. However, this is not necessarily the case and, as with herbal remedies, there is the possibility of poor quality control leading to unexpected effects.

The aim of this book is to evaluate the literature that exists for some of these nutraceuticals and to assess the medical and scientific evidence available. Many chapters originated as articles we previously published in the *Pharmaceutical Journal*. At the outset it was decided to eliminate vitamins and minerals, which are widely reviewed, as well as amino acids as these are well documented elsewhere. The remaining list consists mainly of supplements, which are usually obtained from a food source, but are sold as isolated, purified components in pharmacological doses for specific ailments. The uses and side-effects are described for each one and a general description of nutraceuticals has been included in the introduction.

It is hoped that this work will be useful to pharmacists and medical practitioners, as well as to students associated with the medical professions. Members of the public with an interest in supplemental therapy may also benefit from its information.

Lisa Rapport, Brian Lockwood
September 2001

# Acknowledgements

We would like to acknowledge the continued help of the staff of John Rylands University Library for access to books and periodicals, electronic databases, and rapid supply of Inter Library Loans. BL would also like to thank colleagues for useful conversations and for helping to retain his sanity, and LR would like to thank her understanding husband and children for enabling her to undertake this work.

# About the authors

Brian Lockwood is a practising academic pharmacist who has worked in seven schools of pharmacy and visited many more in the course of his work. He has published many papers and chapters in books in the area of plant medicines, and is a long-standing lecturer to local branches of the Royal Pharmaceutical Society on the subjects of herbal medicine and aromatherapy.

Lisa Rapport is a part-time community pharmacist who in the course of her work has developed a keen interest in complementary therapy and nutritional supplements.

# Abbreviations

**α-KG** alpha ketoglutarate
**ADP** adenosine diphosphate
**ALA** α-linoleic acid
**ALS** amyotrophic lateral sclerosis
**AS** Angelman syndrome
**AZT** zidovudine

**BSA** burn surface area

**$CC_{50}$** concentration necessary to decrease the uptake to 50% of the control
**CHD** coronary heart disease
**CHF** congestive heart failure
**CPAC** proanthocyanidins from *Cupressus sempervirens*
**CSM** Committee on Safety of Medicines
**CVD** cardiovascular disease

**DAO** diamine oxidase
**DFD** defined formula liquid oral diet
**DHA** docosahexaenoic acid
**DNA** deoxyribonucleic acid
**DSHEA** Dietary Supplement Health and Education Act

**$EC_{50}$** 50% effective dose
**ECG** electrocardiogram
**EPA** eicosapentaenoic acid

**FA** fatty acid
**FDA** Food and Drug Administration
**FIM** Foundation for Innovation in Medicine
**5FMOrn** 5-fluoromethylornithine

**GABA** gamma-aminobutyric acid
**GAG** glycosaminoglycan
**GGT** gamma-glutamic transaminase
**GOT** glutamic-oxalacetic transaminase
**GPT** glutamic-pyruvate transaminase
**GSPE** grape seed proanthocyanidin extract

**HCT** haematocrit
**HD** haemodialysis
**HDL-C** high-density lipoprotein cholesterol
**HIV** human immunodeficiency virus
**HPLC** high-performance liquid chromatography
**HRT** hormone replacement therapy
**HTLV** human T lymphotropic virus

**i.m.** intramuscular
**IgA** immunoglobulin A
**IGF-1** insulin-like growth factor
**IL-1β** interleukin 1β
**IL-2** interleukin-2
**ILAR** International League Against Rheumatism

**JHCI** Joint Health Claims Initiative

**LDL-C** low-density lipoprotein cholesterol
**LH** luteinizing hormone
**LT** leukotriene
**$LTB_4$** leukotriene $B_4$
**$LTB_5$** leukotriene $B_5$

**MAOI** monoamine oxidase inhibitor
**MCA** Medicines Control Agency
**MI** myocardial infarction
**MS** mass spectrometry

**NIDDM** non-insulin-dependent diabetes mellitus
**NREA** Nutraceutical Research and Education Act
**NSAID** non-steroidal anti-inflammatory drug

**OA** osteoarthritis
**OAT** ornithine aminotransferase
**ODC** ornithine decarboxylase
**OKG** ornithine alpha ketoglutarate

**PA** polyamine
**PAC** proanthocyanidin
**PAF** platelet-activating factor
**PG** prostaglandin
**$PGE_2$** prostaglandin $E_2$
**$PGE_3$** prostaglandin $E_3$
**$PGH_2$** prostaglandin $H_2$
**PKD** polycystic kidney disease
**PMN** polymorphonuclear neutrophils
**PUFA** polyunsaturated fatty acid

**RA** rheumatoid arthritis
**RBC** red blood cells
**RHuEPO** recombinant human erythropoietin

**SAD** seasonal affective disorder
**SD** secoisolariciresinol-diglycoside
**SLE** systemic lupus erythematosus
**6-SMT** 6-sulfatoxymelatonin

**TLC** thin-layer chromatography
**TNF** tumour necrosis factor
**TPA** 12-*O*-tetradecanoylphorbol-13-acetate
**TPN** total parenteral nutrition
**TX** thromboxane
**$TXA_2$** thromboxane $A_2$
**$TXB_2$** thromboxane $B_2$

**UV** ultraviolet

**VLDL-C** very low-density lipoprotein cholesterol
**VES** vitamin E succinate

**WHO** World Health Organization

# 1

# Introduction

Over the last few years, an increasing number of dietary supplements have become available for self-medication. These are widely available both from pharmacies and from supermarkets and health-food shops, as well as by mail order. This boom in the range and increased availability of supplements has led to increasing interest from the general public and health professionals alike, and the topic is widely discussed by the media.

Many national newspapers devote regular columns to the use of nutritional supplements, and from time to time advertisements or articles in the lay press and especially in women's magazines produce a sudden surge in requests for a particular product. There is also much coverage on the television and radio. Other sources of information on healthy eating and supplements include food packages, health professionals, books, friends and relatives, and leaflets in clinics, schools and colleges.[1]

However, nutrition experts often put forward many conflicting nutritional theories, and these are bound to confuse consumers. One example is the conflict between the recommendation for high-protein, low-carbohydrate versus low-protein, high-carbohydrate versus low-fat diets. Similarly, in the 1970s butter sales were reduced after negative publicity about saturated fats, but since the mid-1990s, polyunsaturated fats (margarine) have been said to be less healthy than saturated fats and *trans* fatty acids have also become an issue, resulting in a resurgence in butter sales.

Often, such changes in the information that consumers receive result in many people ignoring the experts' opinions and making their own decisions.[2] Moreover, while some doctors often recommend alternative therapies, either together with, or instead of conventional medicines, others tell their patients that supplements are unnecessary when the evidence in the medical–nutrition literature clearly advocates their use. To the uninformed this can become very confusing.

## Consumer attitudes to health

In 1998 a survey was carried out by Leatherhead Research Association to assess consumer attitudes to health in three European countries: Britain, France and Germany.[3] The results were based on interviews with 200 housewives in each country and showed how attitudes between countries differ, probably due to information and views that are widespread in that country.

First, the interviewees were asked what criteria they used to judge their own health. In all three countries 'energy levels' came first. 'Absence of illness' came second in France and Germany but third in Britain, where 'physical appearance' came second. Only 9% of British respondents thought cholesterol levels were important, compared with 18% of the French and 32% of the Germans.

When asked which factors motivated the desire to be healthy, 'to feel good' was the reason given most often in all three countries. Other factors varied from country to country including 'to live longer', 'to prevent disease', 'to maintain an active lifestyle' and 'to improve/maintain appearance/weight'.

The women were also asked to rank diet, genetic make-up and exercise in order of importance for health. Diet came first for the British and German respondents, but in France they put exercise first, genetic make-up second and diet third. In Britain, after diet, genetic make-up was thought to be more important than exercise, but in Germany this was reversed.

This survey shows that as a result of the different information available to the public in three European countries, many different opinions prevail and they do not necessarily reflect scientifically proven evidence. It is important that people who are concerned have access to up-to-date and scientifically sound information when making health choices.

## The use of supplements

In a survey carried out by Mintel market research in November 1998,[4] 57% of 979 adults agreed that they would like to use supplements more often, but were unsure of what to buy. This indicated a need for more information.

Market trend surveys carried out by Mintel market research in March 1999,[5] found that the prime target users of supplements were middle-aged females with an above average income and above average education. There were also occasional users who used supplements at a time of illness or stress, rather like a medicine. These users were more varied in age and income and were less likely to take supplements on a long-term basis.

Consumers use supplements for many varied reasons. These include supplementation of a poor diet, to improve overall health, to delay the onset of age-related diseases, after illness, for stress, when recommended by a health professional, in pregnancy and slimming, to improve sports performance and to treat symptoms (colds, coughs, arthritis, etc.).

In America and in Europe the use of alternative medicine, including supplements and nutraceuticals, is increasing. Many theories have been put forward as to why consumers choose alternative over conventional remedies.[6] It is thought that many patients are not satisfied with the treatment they are given by their doctors, either because they experience adverse effects or because the remedy has been ineffective. Another reason for choosing alternative remedies is that patients may feel that conventional medicine is impersonal or technologically orientated. Some patients prefer to have personal control over their health care and therefore are happier to self-select than be told what to take by their doctor. In a survey carried out in America in 1998, a random sample of 1500 patients were included in a mail survey, 1035 (69%) of whom replied (which may have introduced bias as it is possible that people with no interest in alternative therapies did not reply). Forty per cent of those who replied reported using alternative therapies over the previous year. The top four treatments were chiropractic, lifestyle diet, exercise/movement and relaxation. Diet was used mostly for anxiety, chronic fatigue syndrome, muscle sprains/strains, arthritis/rheumatism, depression, digestive problems and diabetes. Results showed that there was no significant difference in alternative treatment users between men and women or income, but higher education did result in increased use. Users also tended to have a holistic philosophy of health, believing in the importance of mind, body and spirit in overall health, but interestingly, users of alternative remedies were no more dissatisfied with conventional therapies than non-users.

## What is a nutraceutical?

Nutraceuticals is a term used to describe medicinally or nutritionally functional foods. They have also been called medical foods, designer foods, phytochemicals, functional foods and nutritional supplements. Nutraceuticals include everyday products such as 'bio' yoghurts and fortified breakfast cereals, as well as vitamins, herbal remedies and even genetically modified foods and supplements. Many terms and definitions are used in different countries and this can become quite confusing.

Dr Stephen De Felice MD, the founder and chairman of the Foundation for Innovation in Medicine (Cranford, NJ, USA), an educational organisation set up in 1976 to encourage medical health research, first coined the term 'nutraceutical' in 1989.[7–9] De Felice defined a nutraceutical as a 'food, or parts of a food, that provide medical or health benefits, including the prevention and treatment of disease'.

In Canada, a functional food has been defined as 'similar in appearance to conventional foods,... consumed as part of a usual diet', whereas a nutraceutical is 'a product produced from foods but sold in pills, powders, (potions) and other medicinal forms not generally associated with food'.[10]

The UK Ministry of Agriculture, Fisheries and Food (now Department for Environment, Food and Rural Affairs) has developed a definition of a functional food as 'a food that has a component incorporated into it to give it a specific medical or physiological benefit, other than purely nutritional benefit'.[11]

Hence, both in Canada and in the UK a 'functional food' is essentially a food, but a 'nutraceutical' is an isolated or concentrated form. In America 'medical foods' and 'dietary supplements' are regulatory terms (see below), but 'nutraceuticals', 'functional foods' and other such terms are determined by consultants and marketers, based on consumer trends.[12]

## Sources of nutraceuticals

Many products promoted to treat various disease states, whether as prescribed medication or as supplements, find their origins in the plant kingdom. This is unsurprising in view of the fact that plants produce many secondary compounds, such as alkaloids, to protect themselves from infection and these constituents are often useful in the treatment of human disease. One example is the recently introduced Taxol, derived from taxoids of the American yew tree and now used in ovarian cancer. Similarly, the role of flavonoids and other plant compounds as antioxidants and free-radical scavengers is beginning to have profound effects in the area of chronic inflammatory disease and cancer.[13]

There is also a long history of plant use in many cultures around the world. These traditional uses can provide clues to identify plants with activity in the treatment of disease.[14] Crude extracts of the different parts of the plant are screened for pharmacological activity, often based on usage in folk medicine. Once a result is found, the substances are identified by chromatography and purified further before *in vivo* testing is started. A few of these lead compounds may eventually become licensed as medicines. However, the main drawback to this process is the vast cost involved.

## Foods or medicines?

In many countries, food labelling regulations do not allow food labels to carry health claims. In the UK, the Joint Health Claims Initiative (JHCI) provides guidance on claims that are allowed for functional foods, such as fortified breakfast cereals and 'bio' yoghurts. In some cases, although medical claims such as 'helps prevent heart disease' are not allowed, health-promoting claims, such as 'helps lower cholesterol' can be made if scientific evidence exists. Many inaccurate claims are, nevertheless, made for many supplements available and it is hardly surprising that Mintel research found that most British consumers were sceptical about health claims and found them misleading.[2] Another cause of confusion is the different units that manufacturers use to express the amount of active substance (international units, micrograms and milligrams).[15]

Companies marketing nutraceuticals cannot advertise the health benefits of their products without a medicine licence; this gives them the choice between either not doing any research at all or spending considerable time and money on researching a new product thoroughly and possibly obtaining a patent. Unfortunately, many companies tend towards the former option due to the costs, the problems of obtaining a patent on a natural product or the fact that they cannot put their claims on the label without a product licence whether verified or not. To bring a medicine to market can take about ten years and cost $250 million, whereas to market an unlicensed nutraceutical takes a fraction of this.[8] An example was the case of Cholestin, a cholesterol-lowering supplement marketed by Pharmanex (Simi Valley, CA, USA) in 1996. This product was made from red yeast rice, a food that has been used for centuries in China. Red yeast rice is made by a natural fermentation process, which generates multiple statins and provides the cholesterol-lowering benefit. When the pharmaceutical company Merck (Whitehouse Station, NJ, USA) tested this supplement, it found that the active ingredient was lovastatin, a known cholesterol-lowering agent available on prescription, which is included in their product Mevacor. In 1998, the US Food and Drug Administration banned Pharmanex from importing red yeast rice for the manufacture of Cholestin on the grounds that one of the many beneficial constituents in red yeast rice is chemically identical to lovastatin. As can be seen from this example, the difference between pharmaceutical and nutraceutical is sometimes difficult to define, depending only on regulatory issues. However, in February 1999, a district court ruled that Cholestin was indeed a dietary supplement, based on the US Dietary Supplement Health and Education Act of 1994 and Cholestin remains available in its original form.[16,17]

In the UK, there are four different legal categories of herbal remedies:

- Prescription-only herbal remedies with a product licence.
- Pharmacy-only herbal remedies with a product licence.
- General sale list herbal remedies with a product licence.
- Herbal remedies exempt from licensing and marketed as food supplements and cosmetics.

Depending on issues such as health claims, presentation and dosage, a particular substance can be classed as either a food or a medicine. There are also a vast number of products in a borderline area;[18] these substances would include nutraceuticals and need classification as medicines, foods or some other category. In the UK, unlicensed herbal remedies and supplements are marketed without medical claims and as such are legally regarded as food supplements controlled by the Department for Environment, Food and Rural Affairs. However, they can still be presented as a medicine with regard to packaging and recommended dose, which can confuse the public. In the past, as long as the products did not claim to have medicinal uses, the Medicines Control Agency (MCA), the body that is responsible for regulating medicinal products, did not require that the product satisfied medical legislation.[19] However, more emphasis is now being placed on the *function* of the marketed product as Britain moves in line with the rest of Europe. It was recently reported that the control of herbal products is to move to the European Commission[20] and it is likely that supplements will follow a similar course. Article 1 of Directive 65/65 EEC[21] defines a medicinal product as 'any substance or combination of substances presented for treating, or preventing disease in human beings or animals' and 'any substance or combination of substances which may be administered to human beings or animals with a view to making diagnosis or to restoring, correcting or modifying physiological functions in human beings or animals is likewise considered a medicinal product.' The second definition describes a product that has a medical function irrespective of whether these claims have been stated or not; this would include many supplements being taken for medical purposes.

British licensed medicines for human use are regulated according to the Medicines Act 1968[22] and the Medicines for Human Use (Marketing Authorisations etc.) Regulations 1994 SI3144 (The Regulations).[23] In 1995 these regulations came into effect implementing all the controls as listed in Directive 65/65 EEC. According to these regulations there are controls over variation and renewal of UK licences as well as labelling and package inserts.

In the USA, a new product may be eligible for regulatory status as a food, a dietary supplement or as a medical food.[24] The US Congress passed the Dietary Supplement Health and Education Act (DSHEA) in 1994. This set up a new regulatory body for dietary supplements under the US Food and Drug Administration (FDA). Unlike foods, dietary supplements are allowed to use 'nutritional support statements'. These may offer nutritional support in nutrient-deficiency disease, or state a description of the intended role, mechanism of action or effect on general health as a result of taking the product. For those dietary supplements for which such a statement is used the label must also state: 'This statement has not been evaluated by the Food and Drug Administration. This product is not intended to diagnose, treat, cure or prevent any disease.' In effect, because legally they are in a class by themselves, dietary supplements in the US can be marketed without the FDA being satisfied that they are safe. This makes it relatively easy for a manufacturer to market a product without investing the time and money required for its safety.

Dr De Felice and the Foundation for Innovation in Medicine (FIM) is involved in promoting public awareness of nutraceuticals and ensuring that the results of clinical trials, rather than the business market, drive the nutraceutical industry.[25,26] The FIM introduced the Nutraceutical Research and Education Act (NREA) in Congress on 1 October 1999.[27] This Act proposes the promotion of clinical research and development of dietary supplements and foods for their health benefits (nutraceuticals) and the establishment of a new legal classification to give exclusive rights to the company doing the research for a set time period.

Of all three categories – food, dietary supplement and medical food – medical foods have the least formal regulatory controls. In 1990, US Congress defined a medical food as: 'a food which is formulated to be consumed or administered enterally under the supervision of a physician and which is intended for the specific dietary management of a disease or condition for which distinctive nutritional requirements, based on recognised scientific principles, are established by medical evaluation.'[24] These products are usually promoted through health-care professionals, including pharmacists, and in the UK this would make them prescription-only or pharmacy medicines.

## Quality assurance

Medicines are subject to strict quality control, including the testing of disintegration, bioavailability and precise amounts of active ingredients.[15] Although some manufacturers carry out their own tests, others do not due to the cost involved.

Some supplements are sold in 'standardised' amounts, where the manufacturer has determined that there is the same amount of active ingredient in each preparation, but others are rather haphazard. For example, in a study to determine the actual contents of 14 glucosamine preparations and 11 chondroitin sulfate preparations it was found that the amounts often differed significantly from those stated on the labels, with variations as a low as 0% and as high as 115%.[28] There is also much variation in the actual products, depending on storage, manufacturing process or even which batch of a material is tested. It is vital that these discrepancies are resolved, possibly with the creation of a third type of regulatory category for supplements,[27] as has been suggested in America by De Felice.

## Safety

A five-year study of side-effects of traditional remedies, herbal remedies and dietary supplements was carried out between 1991 and 1995 in the Medical Toxicology Unit at Guys' Hospital, London.[29] Of the 1297 enquiries assessed (23% of all enquiries) an association from 'possible' to 'confirmed' was made in 61% of cases. These included allergic reactions, gastrointestinal symptoms and liver function abnormalities (mainly from Chinese herbal medicines), as well as potential interactions between self-prescribed supplementary remedies and prescribed medication. The authors concluded that the overall risk factor with these products was low and that they were generally considered to be safe. Many of these products are self-prescribed and consumers assume that what is natural is safe, which may lead to inappropriate use, overdose or interactions with other medications. Also, because many health-care professionals considered these products as little more than placebo, side-effects were often not traced back to the supplements being used, either because the patient did not tell their doctor they were taking the supplements or because the doctor did not report the supplement as a possible cause of the side-effect/interaction.

This study highlights the importance of research in this area. Many consumers are unaware of the difference between licensed and unlicensed products or the differences between food legislation and medicine legislation. Pharmacists in the UK are now being encouraged to use the Yellow Card Scheme, run by the Medicines Control Agency (MCA) on behalf of the Committee on Safety of Medicines (CSM), to report suspected drug reactions from both unlicensed and licensed supplements as well as conventional medicines. This scheme relies on health professionals reporting side-effects they suspect to be related to the medicine a patient is taking. Another important conclusion of the project is the need to increase awareness among medical professionals of the use of supplements by their patients and to improve the provision of information about supplements to health-care professionals.

Over the last 20 years or so, there has been a revolution in dietary supplements and many members of the public are seeking to improve their health either through diet or through 'natural' remedies. It cannot be overemphasised that whilst many components of foods may be safe at the normal levels of intake, once these levels are increased to 'pharmacological' levels, other effects may appear. It is therefore imperative that these nutraceuticals are properly researched and that health professionals, as well as the public, are well-informed of the benefits and drawbacks of these medications.

## Evidence from trials

In order to provide conclusive evidence of the role of a particular nutraceutical either in preventing or in treating disease, several factors are needed. First, an inverse relationship between body levels of the supplement and risk of disease must be shown and the levels required must be established. Research teams use many different types of evaluation. Unfortunately, many of these have significant drawbacks. For example, animal studies are often used, but although these may give conclusive results, they may be irrelevant to humans. Another method is the use of *in vitro* studies, looking at cell and tissue responses in isolation; these may well produce results quite different from the response of that tissue when exposed *in vivo*. They also do not take into account the effect of absorption of the substance after digestion. Epidemiological studies are another widely used type of investigation. For example, it has been shown that Japanese women who consume soya in large amounts suffer very little from sex-hormone-related cancers compared with Western women who have very little soya products in their diet.[30] Although such small-scale human studies are popular with researchers, it is maintained by many in the field that only large clinical trials can provide conclusive evidence for the effect of nutraceuticals in the prevention and treatment of disease.[3]

## Using clinical trials

When studying a nutraceutical for its disease-preventing properties, such as antioxidants used to prevent the development of atherosclerosis or cancer, ideally a healthy human population should be studied until sufficient numbers have developed the disease. This is obviously impractical and would require a very large population over a very long time. Therefore researchers resort to studying subjects who already have the disease or who are at high risk of developing the disease.[3] It is assumed that if high-risk or diseased patients are cured, then healthy subjects would benefit from the supplement in question as a preventative measure. But just because high-risk patients are cured, can it be assumed that healthy patients will also derive benefit? Moreover, if high-risk or diseased patients are not helped, does this mean that healthy subjects will not derive benefit either?

There is another important factor to consider when carrying out clinical trials for nutraceuticals. Whereas with drugs it can be safely assumed that the subject is receiving no other source of the test substance, a nutraceutical is often a pharmacological dose of a substance that is present in much smaller amounts in the normal diet or in the body (e.g. melatonin). This makes it very difficult to assess the baseline levels of the placebo group, which may vary considerably between subjects, depending on the time of day or the diet.

In her book, *Handbook of Dietary Supplements*, Mason asserts that a combination of several types of double-blind trials is required to evaluate any particular supplement:[15]

- Cross-cultural epidemiological studies must show any association between low levels of the nutrient in a sample population and high levels of disease.
- In the same study group there must be a relationship between low initial levels of the nutrient and subsequent high risk for the disease.
- Supplementation of the nutrient to a sample population must show a reduced incidence of the disease, compared with a group that receives only placebo.

An illustration of how the wrong conclusions can sometimes be reached because researchers have failed to consider all possibilities is provided by the case of betacarotene. In 1981, epidemiological data suggested that betacarotene may reduce the risk of cancer.[31] However, in 1994 and 1996, two studies were published in which long-term smokers or asbestos workers showed an increased risk of cancer after prolonged supplementation with betacarotene .[32,33] Subsequently it was shown that several important errors had been made first in promoting betacarotene as an effective anti-cancer agent and then in scares that it increased the risk of cancer.[34] First, synthetic betacarotene was assumed to work in the same way as the natural supplement, although it is now known that the two isomers have different stereochemistry. Moreover, although previous studies did not indicate that betacarotene was useful in lung cancer, this was the population that the researchers chose to study. The dietary supplements were also given at a late stage of cancer progression; this does not rule out the possibility of its benefit if used in the early phases of cancer development.[35] Also, the researchers concentrated on betacarotene because it was easy to study, but did not take into account the possibility that it was masking other carotenoids in foods. It was also not considered that carotenoids act together rather than as separate entities. Many supplements originating in foods are not pharmaceuticals that work as magic bullets, but rather act synergistically by interacting with the many micronutrients present. Indeed, the disease-preventing properties of betacarotene remain strong, but only when used in conjunction with other carotenoids that complement its action.[34]

## Summary

This chapter has given an overview of consumer attitudes to nutraceuticals and other supplements, as well as describing the different definitions of nutraceuticals according to the regulations in several countries. Moreover, the types of trials required to provide clinical evidence for their use has also been outlined. In the following chapters, the individual nutraceuticals chosen will be reviewed separately and the results and implications of the research published to date will be reported.

## References

1. Shortt C. Communicating the benefits of functional foods to the consumer. In: Buttriss J, Saltmarsh M, eds. *Functional Foods II, Claims and Evidence*. Cambridge, UK: The Royal Society of Chemistry; 2000: 70–74.

2. *Mintel Market Intelligence*, Functional Foods, March 2000.
3. Young J. Functional foods and the European consumer. In: Buttriss J, Saltmarsh M, eds. *Functional Foods II, Claims and Evidence*. Cambridge, UK: The Royal Society of Chemistry, 2000: 75–78.
4. *Mintel Market Intelligence*, Complementary Medicines, March 1999: 1–38.
5. *Mintel Market Intelligence*, Functional Foods, March 1999: 1–47.
6. Asin J A. Why patients use alternative medicine, results of a national study. *JAMA* 1998; 279: 1548–1553.
7. Jack D B. Keep taking the tomatoes – the exciting world of nutraceuticals, *Mol Med Today* 1995; 118–121.
8. Brower B. Nutraceuticals: Poised for a healthy slice of the market. *Nature Biotechnol* 1998; 16: 728–733.
9. Mannion M. Nutraceutical revolution continues at Foundation for Innovation in Medicine Conference. *Am J Nat Med* 1998; 5: 30–33.
10. Mazza G. *Functional Foods*. Pennsylvania: Technomic Publishing, 1998.
11. Cockbill C A. Food law and functional foods. *Br Food J* 1994; 96: 3–4.
12. Aarts T A. How long will the 'Medical Food' window of opportunity remain open? *J Nutraceuticals Function Med Foods* 1998; 1: 45–57.
13. Anon. Pharmaceuticals from plants: great potential, few funds. *Lancet* 1994; 343: 1513.
14. Senior K. Pharmaceuticals from plants: promise and progress. *Mol Med Today* 1996; 60–64.
15. Mason P. *Handbook of Dietary Supplements*. Oxford: Blackwell Science, 1995.
16. Morrow P R, Pharmanex, Inc. Private correspondence, 2001.
17. Heber D, Yip I, Ashley J M, *et al.* Cholesterol-lowering effects of a proprietary Chinese red-yeast-rice dietary supplement. *Am J Clin Nutr* 1999; 69: 231–236.
18. Mason P. The regulation of herbal products in Europe – from diversity to harmonisation? *Pharm J* 2000; 264: 856–857.
19. Newall C A, Anderson L A, Phillipson J D. *Herbal Medicines*. London: Pharmaceutical Press, 1996.
20. Anon. Herbal medicines controls move to Europe. *Pharm J* 1999; 263: 775.
21. Council Directive 65/65/EEC. *Off J EC* 1965; 22: 369.
22. The Medicines Act, 1968. London: HM Stationery Office.
23. Statutory Instrument (SI) 1994:3144, The Medicines for Human Use (Marketing Authorisations etc) Regulations.
24. Litov R E. Developing claims for new phytochemical products. In: Bidlack W R, Omaye S T, Meskin M S, *et al.* eds. *Phytochemicals. A New Paradigm*. Pennsylvania: Technomic Publishing, 1998: 173–176.
25. Foundation for Innovation in Medicine (FIM). www.fimdefelice.org (accessed 1 September 2001).
26. Mannion M. The current nutraceutical health sector and the next phase of the nutraceutical revolution. www.fimdefelice.org/summary11.html (accessed 1 September 2001).
27. The Nutraceutical Research and Education Act. Bill H.R.3001. www.fimdefelice.org/arc.nrea.html (accessed 1 September 2001).
28. Eddington N D. Quality assurance of nutraceuticals in marketed products and

raw materials: case study with chondroitin and glucosamine content in products and permeability across Caco-2 cells. Pharmacokinetics-Biopharmaceutics Laboratory, University of Maryland, Baltimore, MD, USA. Abstract Paper – Am Chem Soc 2000, 220th AGFD-149. CODEN:ACSRAL ISSN:0065-7727. Journal; Meeting abstract written in English. AN 2000: 793181.

29. Shaw D, Leon C, Kolev S, *et al.* Traditional remedies and food supplements, a 5-year toxicological study. *Drug Safety* 1997; 17: 342–356.
30. Mason P. Isoflavones. *Pharm J* 2001; 266: 16–19.
31. Peto R, Doll R, Buckley J D, *et al.* Can dietary beta-carotene materially reduce human cancer rates? *Nature* 1981; 280: 201–208.
32. The Alpha Tocopherol, Beta-carotene Cancer Prevention Study Group. The effects of vitamin E and β-carotene on the incidence of lung cancer and other cancers in male smokers. *N Engl J Med* 1994; 330: 1029–1035.
33. Omenn G S, Goodman G E, Thornquist M D, *et al.* Effects of a combination of β-carotene and vitamin A on lung cancer and cardiovascular disease. *N Engl J Med* 1996; 334: 1150–1155.
34. Challem J J. Beta-carotene and other carotenoids: promises, failures, and a new vision. *J Orthomol Med* 1997; 12: 11–19.
35. Astorg P, Gradelet S, Berges R, *et al.* Dietary lycopene decreases the initiation of liver preneoplastic foci by diethylnitrosamine in the rat. *Nutr Cancer* 1997; 29: 60–68.

# 2

# Glucosamine

A survey carried out by the Department of Complementary Medicine at the University of Exeter, UK, in 1993 found that there was wide public interest in complementary medicines for arthritis sufferers.[1] It was found that fish oil and evening primrose oil were used most often, with fish oil being perceived as most helpful. From the study, it could be seen that many arthritis sufferers were not satisfied with their conventional treatments and they therefore looked for alternative options that would alleviate symptoms with few adverse effects. Glucosamine is a nutraceutical that could fill these requirements. It is available from health-food shops, from pharmacies and via the Internet.

## Properties and structure

Glucosamine is an amino-monosaccharide made up of glucose and the amino acid glutamic acid (Figure 2.1).[2] It is found naturally in the body and is present in almost all human tissue, especially in cartilage, tendons and ligament tissues, where it has an important role as a precursor of the disaccharide units of articular cartilage glycosaminoglycan (GAG).[2,3] Glucosamine has a molecular weight of just 179 and because it is such a small molecule it is absorbed very easily and is taken up preferentially by cartilage and other joint structures.[4–6] The sulfate form, which is still a small compound, is usually used for therapeutic purposes.

Glucosamine is not found in significant amounts in the usual diet and must be synthesised by the body. This ability declines with age and predisposes the body to degenerative joint disease or arthritis.

## Glucosamine as a treatment for arthritis

Osteoarthritis (OA, also called osteoarthrosis) and rheumatic arthritis (RA) are more commonly found in women than in men, with 1% of the adult population suffering from RA and 10% of the elderly (over 65) having symptoms of OA. This prevalence in the elderly makes arthritis

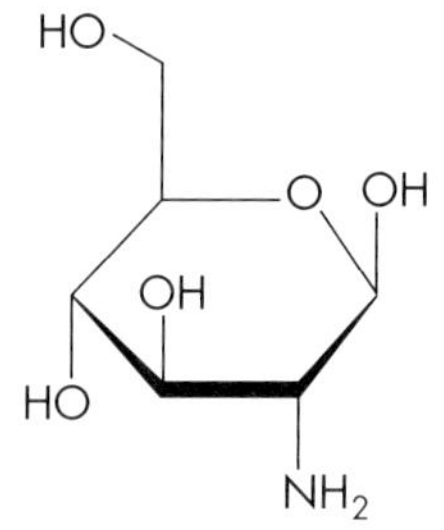

**Figure 2.1** Structure of glucosamine.

almost a normal part of ageing. Although the two can coexist, OA and RA have different symptoms and are managed differently.[6,7]

OA is a slowly progressive disease, which affects the joints of the hips and knees, but can also affect the hands and spine. Initially it is a non-inflammatory disease and due to changes in the biochemical composition of the articular cartilage there is decreased elasticity, leading to degeneration and functional deterioration of the joint. Since the cartilage protects the joint by a shock-absorbing and cushioning effect, cartilage degeneration gradually leads to the loss of joint function.[2] Secondary to this process, inflammation occurs due to the increased release of inflammatory mediators, and osteophytes (bone protrusions) may result, causing enlarged joints, pain on activity and immobility. Surgical joint replacement may be required if there is major disability.

RA is an inflammatory condition affecting multiple joints of the hands, wrists and elbows. It may be autoimmune or genetic. The synovium around the joint is infiltrated with B and T lymphocytes and macrophages, resulting in destruction of the joint. The pain that ensues is present even at rest and the joints are tender and swollen.

The two main aims in treating arthritis patients are management of the symptoms, mainly pain and movement limitation, and slowing the disease process.[3] Glucosamine seems to do both and therefore could be an agent of choice. At present its effects have only been researched in OA, where cartilage damage is the cause of the condition.

## How does it work?

### *Chondroprotection*

Chondroprotection is the term used when exogenous GAGs are used to synthesise proteoglycans. GAGs have also been shown to have an anti-inflammatory effect.[8] Glucosamine is such a chondroprotective agent and is often used in conjunction with a second agent, chondroitin sulfate.

D-Glucosamine, the active principle of glucosamine sulfate, is a small molecule that readily diffuses through all biological membranes. It has a high affinity for cartilaginous tissue, and is incorporated into proteoglycan molecules. As stated above, it is a preferred building block for the synthesis of GAGs, and these offer protection against the cartilage-damaging effects of non-steroidal anti-inflammatory drugs (NSAIDs) and steroids. Glucosamine also inhibits the release of proteolytic enzymes and lysosomal enzymes, but not by the inhibition of prostaglandin biosynthesis, which is responsible for the anti-inflammatory actions of NSAIDs. Thus glucosamine is anti-arthritic and anti-inflammatory and acts against joint degeneration as well as offering joint protection.[6,8]

The enzyme elastase plays an important role in the breakdown of the articular cartilage, ligaments, tendons and bones in RA and it has been shown that *N*-acetylglucosamine mildly inhibits elastase in a dose-dependent way. *N*-Acetylglucosamine may therefore modify the disease processes of RA as well as of OA.[9]

Glucosamine shows long-term disease-modifying activity and its effects are only seen after several weeks of therapy. It has therefore been proposed that it should be classified as a drug to be included in the subcategory 'slow acting drugs in osteoarthritis' by the International League Against Rheumatism (ILAR). This difference in kinetics is related to the different mechanisms of action of glucosamine when compared with NSAIDs.[3]

### *The hexosamine pathway*

Endogenous glucosamine is a product of the hexosamine pathway, which is involved in insulin responses. Experiments have shown that glucosamine can induce insulin resistance via this pathway, without the presence of high glucose concentration, and that fat-induced insulin resistance is likewise affected by the presence of glucosamine.[10] Thus glucosamine can cause 'glucose toxicity', which worsens the diabetic state and makes regulation more difficult, leading to the defects in insulin secretion seen in non-insulin-dependent diabetes mellitus (NIDDM).[11] In the normal state, blood concentrations of glucosamine are negligible, but when the body is exposed to non-physiological concentrations of glucosamine, this hexosamine pathway appears to be activated, leading to changes in glucose utilisation. A recent study investigated the effect of glucosamine on insulin secretion and action in ten healthy males.[12] It found that an infusion of glucosamine increased glucose utilisation and caused a mild dysfunction of insulin β-cells, most probably via the hexosamine pathway. This led to a decreased glucose tolerance.

As osteoarthritis patients are often elderly and obese and at high risk for NIDDM, this effect is possibly of great significance and points to the need for very large-scale clinical trials.

## Methods of administration

Glucosamine has been used to treat osteoarthritis for more than 20 years. In a double-blind study in an Italian hospital in 1980, its effects were compared with placebo.[13] Eighty patients were given two capsules of glucosamine 250 mg or placebo three times daily, before meals. The intensity of symptoms such as pain, joint tenderness and swelling were recorded each week for a month. At the end of the treatment period, significantly more of the glucosamine patients were pain-free and some were totally symptom-free, the reduction in symptoms being twice as large and twice as fast as that in the patients taking placebo. In a few patients taking part in this study, cartilage samples were required for other reasons (after accidents or due to surgery). These were examined using electron microscopy and it was found that in those patients receiving glucosamine the articular cartilage seemed to have been rebuilt. More research was required than was possible using this very small sample of patients, but these results were very encouraging. In addition, this trial was only one month in duration, which is short for glucosamine treatment, and so neither the long-term benefits nor side-effects were noted.[6]

Another early trial was carried out using arthritis patients in Thailand, where because of their usual sitting position, OA of the knee, or gonarthrosis, is a major problem and prevents many people from working and functioning normally.[14] The double-blind study using 54 patients compared intra-articular glucosamine with a normal saline placebo. Each patient received a weekly injection in the affected knee for five weeks (dose not specified) and results were noted a month after the end of the treatment period. Exercise, a reduced-calorie diet and avoidance of acute flexion, extension and loading of the knee were recommended for the duration of the study. Both treatments significantly decreased pain and increased the ability to climb five steps, but the glucosamine resulted in more pain-free patients. The improvement with glucosamine, however, also lasted for at least the following month. There was partial articular function return and effective relief of pain. No side-effects were reported for either group.

A larger double-blind study was carried out to determine the effects of intramuscular (i.m.) glucosamine versus placebo.[4] One hundred and fifty-five patients with chronic gonarthrosis symptoms were recruited for the study from ten outpatient clinics. They were randomly divided to receive twice-weekly i.m. injections of either 400 mg glucosamine sulfate or placebo (normal saline) for six weeks. All other OA treatments were stopped for the duration of the study except for paracetamol for unbearable pain. Results showed a significant improvement of symptoms in the glucosamine group compared with placebo, and this improvement increased as the trial progressed. Tolerability of glucosamine was not different from that of placebo with around 5% incidence of minor side-effects (nausea, headache, skin reactions and local reactions).

Although injectable preparations proved useful, especially when the OA was very localised as in the examples above, since glucosamine is well absorbed by the oral route, the availability of 500-mg tablets made evaluation simple and introduced the possibility of long-term therapy.[15]

There has been one long-term study carried out recently on the effects of glucosamine on OA progression.[16] This was a randomised, double-blind, placebo-controlled trial. All patients were over 50 years of age, and suffered from OA of the knee. Two hundred and twelve patients were randomly assigned to receive either 1500 mg glucosamine or placebo, once daily for three years. There was a similar drop-out rate in the two groups over the three years, with similar reasons given. Although symptoms in the placebo group worsened, there was a significant improvement in symptoms in the test group. Joint-space width was also measured and was found to be progressively narrowing in the placebo group, but not in the test group. This suggests that glucosamine not only acts as a symptom-modifying agent but also a structure-modifying agent. Adverse effect reporting was similar in the two groups and laboratory tests showed no metabolic changes, including no changes in glucose metabolism.

## Comparison with conventional treatments

The most widely used class of drugs for OA is the non-steroidal anti-inflammatory drugs (NSAIDs), which are very commonly prescribed by a doctor or bought over the counter to alleviate the pain and other symptoms associated with arthritic conditions. The most commonly used NSAIDs are aspirin, ibuprofen, naproxen, diclofenac and indometacin. Although the mode of action has not been completely elucidated for all NSAIDs, it is accepted that inhibition of prostaglandin synthesis is the mechanism involved.[8]

Even though generally thought to be safe, NSAIDs can have serious side-effects such as gastrointestinal ulcers, which are often not detected until the symptoms have progressed to a serious level. Even short courses of NSAIDs have been shown to cause gastric surface epithelial damage and long-term use can result in hospitalisation and serious damage.[8]

Both the useful and the harmful effects of NSAIDs are related to the prostaglandin synthesis inhibition. A recent study has shown that as well as the well-documented gastrointestinal effects seen with NSAIDs, an additional risk is the development of congestive heart failure (CHF) in certain individuals.[17] The elderly are at increased risk and it is this population that are most commonly prescribed this class of medication for arthritic diseases. The authors of this study found that the use of NSAIDs increased the chances of being admitted to hospital with CHF, although this may have been due to acceleration of a potential condition. Overall, the evidence suggests that NSAIDs should be used with caution in the elderly and in those with a predisposition to CHF and long-term use is best avoided.

Another complication associated with the widespread use of NSAIDs is that they have been shown to cause 'analgesic arthropathy', thought to result either from a loss of pain sensation or from a direct action of the drug on the cartilage, causing a rapid deterioration of the joints.[8]

In an attempt to find an alternative to this class of drugs to avoid the many harmful effects that result in their use, several studies have compared the use of glucosamine with NSAIDs. A double-blind study comparing glucosamine with ibuprofen was carried out in 1982.[18] Forty outpatients with OA of the knee were included and received either 500 mg glucosamine or 400 mg ibuprofen three times daily with meals for eight weeks. Although pain decreased in both groups, in the ibuprofen group there was a sharp decrease for two weeks, which levelled off, whereas in the glucosamine group pain decreased much more slowly but continued for the entire trial period, reaching a lower score after eight weeks. Side-effects were similar in both groups. The authors therefore suggested a possible treatment using a combination of ibuprofen and glucosamine for an initial two weeks, followed by continuation with glucosamine alone.

More recently, a similar but much larger study showed that 500 mg glucosamine compared favourably with 400 mg ibuprofen when both were given orally three times a day for four weeks.[3] Two hundred patients suffering from painful, chronic gonarthrosis took part, most between 50 and 65 years of age. The study was run as a randomised, double-blind, parallel-group design in two different clinics. All other medication for OA was stopped for the duration of the trial, but physical therapy was continued. Medication for other diseases was allowed but had to be registered.

Although the overall results were similar in both groups, the ibuprofen produced a relief of pain almost immediately, whereas the full effect of the glucosamine was seen after two weeks of treatment. There were far more side-effects noted in the ibuprofen group, most being gastrointestinal, but skin reactions were also noted. This led to seven drop-outs. In the glucosamine group side-effects were reported in only six patients and only one dropped out, which is comparable with other studies, where it did not differ from placebo. This difference in adverse effects and drop-outs is significant. If a treatment causes patients to stop taking it then the treatment has failed, which is worth considering when selecting a treatment regimen for a particular patient. Even if the therapy has very good predicted results, it can only achieve these if the patient is compliant. Even though both therapies led to the same control of symptoms, glucosamine had more chance of success due to the possibility of non-compliance in the ibuprofen group because of the side-effects.

Animal studies have been carried out to compare indometacin, another widely used NSAID, with glucosamine.[19] In models of subacute inflammation in rats, glucosamine was found to be 10–30 times safer and therefore more suitable in long-term therapy than indometacin, which caused serious damage to the gastrointestinal tract.

## Dose

A usual recommended dose for glucosamine is 500 mg three times daily. Tablets containing 750 mg are also obtainable for a twice-daily regimen, making compliance easier. Anecdotal evidence has shown that after a few months of taking 500 mg three times daily, the effects were maintained when the dose was reduced to 500 mg twice daily.[8] Often chondroitin sulfate, which is a glycoaminoglycan synthesised by chondrocytes, is taken with glucosamine. Tablets incorporating both supplements are available.

## Side-effects and contraindications

Since glucosamine is a natural constituent of the human body, it has very little toxicity.[8] A large, nationwide study carried out in Portugal involved 252 doctors reporting on 1506 arthrosis outpatients, of whom 1208 completed the study.[20] The trial lasted from September 1980 to May 1981 over the winter months when most cases of arthritis are diagnosed. Each patient received two capsules of glucosamine sulfate 250 mg three times a day for six to eight weeks. Scores were recorded by the doctor for pain (at rest, on standing and on exercise) and mobility before the start of treatment, after two weeks, after three to four weeks and after six to eight weeks. Recordings were also taken in the period from two to twelve weeks after the end of treatment. The overall results were classed as 'good' for 58.7%, 'sufficient' for 36% and 'insufficient' for 5.3% of patients. Of the latter group a third had not responded to previous treatments either.

As might be expected in any large group of patients, many suffered from other diseases in addition to arthrosis and were taking medication for various complaints. The most common additional complaint was cardiovascular disease (24.7%), followed by gastroduodenal problems (8.6%), diabetes (7.6%), hepatic disease (4.9%) and obesity (2.2%). Medications being used included antihypertensives, antacids and anti-ulcer drugs, oral hypoglycaemics and diuretics. A different statistical distribution was noted in patients with obesity and gastroduodenal problems compared with those without other illnesses. In the case of obesity, this may be explained by the fact that the condition is an aggravating factor in arthritis, as well as which, obese patients may need a dose adjustment. For patients suffering from gastroduodenal disorders, the reason may be that they are less likely to take the full oral dose all the time. Diuretics also had an effect on the treatment and again a dose change may be required.

Overall, 186 side-effects were noted in 146 patients. It was impossible to know whether these complaints were due to other illnesses, other medication or the glucosamine treatment. Other treatments were being used in 36% of patients with no side-effects and in 54% of patients with side-effects. All side-effects were reversible and most were gastrointestinal.

The authors concluded that glucosamine is a useful treatment in arthritis, combining efficacy and tolerability. The presence of other illnesses or treatments did not influence the efficacy or tolerability of the glucosamine except in a few cases.

In another paper,[21] a Canadian doctor who had treated over 300 patients with glucosamine reported only one minor side-effect of nausea. He also reported that as a consequence of the positive results experienced by his patients, many started giving glucosamine to their dogs with such good effects that vets in the area have adopted glucosamine as a standard treatment for osteoarthritic pets!

Other citations quote side-effects in the region of 5–6%, most of which are gastrointestinal in nature and can be reduced by taking glucosamine with food.[3,22]

## Flaws in methodology

These studies have been criticised for being too short.[23] The recommendations from a task force of the Osteoarthritis Research Society[24] state that for symptom-modifying drugs where the effect is seen several weeks after the start of therapy (as in the case of glucosamine) 'trials will vary from 3–12 months in length.... Longer trials (up to 2 years) may be required to exclude toxicity or establish long-term benefit.' Many studies described in the literature were much shorter than this and therefore long-term conclusions cannot be made. Consultants who subscribe to *Medical Letters*[25] also found the published trials 'unconvincing' for this reason.

Some trials have been criticised for comparing a maximum dose of 500 mg glucosamine three times daily to half the maximum dose of NSAIDs. For example, 400 mg ibuprofen three times daily was used in the studies described in references 3 and 18.[23] These doses were probably chosen to reduce the NSAID side-effects, but it is true that an unfair comparison was being made.

A meta-analysis of controlled, double-blind, randomised trials of longer than four weeks has been carried out to assess the validity of the clinical trials of glucosamine and chondroitin.[26,27] Many published studies did not satisfy these criteria and were therefore not included in the study. Fifteen trials were analysed, including eight that referred to glucosamine. The authors concluded from their analysis that although glucosamine does have a place in the treatment of arthritic conditions for limited time periods (three months has been suggested[28]), many studies have reported exaggerated effects. These may have been due to methodological flaws or publication bias (trials with significant results are more likely to be published). This emphasises the need for good, scientific research for nutraceuticals, as many claims are made for the benefits of these supplements without sufficient evidence.

## Conclusions

Glucosamine provides a progressive and gradual decline in articular pain and also improves mobility. It is important to remind patients that the effects take time and therefore combined therapy (with analgesics or NSAIDs) may be necessary for the first few weeks of treatment.[6]

Having said that, vigilance is required, as very few long-term studies have been carried out on glucosamine. Overweight patients as well as those with diabetes should be warned to exercise caution before starting treatment, due to possible interference with glucose control. Also, as it is an unlicensed product, obtaining supplies from a reputable company will ensure the quality of the glucosamine. Several quality-assurance studies have found that the amount stated on the label is not necessarily the amount present in the product.[29,30] Moreover, although glucosamine hydrochloride is widely available, most published reports have used the sulfate. One recent study[31] investigated the efficacy of glucosamine hydrochloride for pain in OA of the knee. It was found that there was no significant difference in pain reduction between glucosamine hydrochloride and placebo when measured by a total osteoarthritis index (with scores for pain stiffness and function), although the secondary endpoint of pain reduction by daily diary and knee examination was more favourable. The hydrochloride salt therefore seems to be less effective than the sulfate, but more trials are required.

From the literature searched, it seems that glucosamine is a safe, effective and well-tolerated alternative to NSAIDs in the treatment of degenerative joint disease, with no significant side-effects in short-term use, as well as sustained effects after withdrawal. Many OA patients are prescribed long-term NSAIDs for their condition. These are not ideal for all patients and may lead to severe gastrointestinal effects. Added to this, NSAIDs may accelerate joint deterioration and so in treating the symptoms they worsen the disease. Glucosamine therefore seems a promising alternative. Although studies have concentrated on OA, it would be interesting to consider whether benefits are also seen in other types of arthritis.

## References

1. Ernst E. Over-the-counter complementary remedies used for arthritis. *Pharm J* 1998; 260: 830–831.
2. Briffa J. Glucosamine sulphate in the treatment of osteoarthritis. *Int J Altern Complement Med* 1997; 15: 15–16.

3. Muller-Fabbender H, Bach G L, Haase W, *et al.* Glucosamine sulphate compared to ibuprofen in osteoarthritis of the knee. *Osteoarthritis Cartilage* 1994; 2: 61–69.
4. Reichelt A, Forster K K, Fischer M, *et al.* Efficacy and safety of intramuscular glucosamine sulfate in osteoarthritis of the knee. *Arzneim-Forsch/Drug Res* 1994; 44: 75–79.
5. Webb M. Glucosamine sulphate: superior to NSAIDs in arthritic conditions. *JAMA* 1995; 13: 13.
6. Da Camara C C, Dowless G V. Glucosamine sulfate for osteoarthritis. *Ann Pharmacother* 1998; 32: 580–587.
7. Krska J. The treatment of arthritic conditions. *Pharmacy Mag* 2000; 6: 17–25.
8. Gottleib M S. Conservative management of spinal osteoarthritis with glucosamine sulfate and chiropractic treatment. *J Manipulative Physiol Ther* 1997; 20: 400–414.
9. Kamel M, Hanafi M, Bassiouni M. Inhibition of elastase enzyme release from human polymorphonuclear leukocytes by N-acetyl-galactosamine and N-acetyl-glucosamine. *Clin Exp Rheum* 1991; 9: 17–21.
10. Hussain M A. A case for glucosamine. *Eur J Endocrinol* 1998; 139: 472–475.
11. McClain D A, Crook E D. Hexamines and insulin resistance. *Diabetes* 1996; 45: 1003–1009.
12. Monauni T, Zenti M G, Cretti A, *et al.* Effects of glucosamine infusion on insulin secretion and insulin action in humans. *Diabetes* 2000; 49: 926–935.
13. Drovanti A, Bignamini A A, Rovati A L. Therapeutic activity of oral glucosamine sulfate in osteoarthritis. *Clin Ther* 1980; 3: 260–272.
14. Vajaradul Y. Double-blind clinical evaluation of intra articular glucosamine in out-patients with gonarthrosis. *Clin Ther* 1981; 3: 336–343.
15. McCarty M F. The neglect of glucosamine as a treatment for osteoarthritis – a personal perspective. *Med Hypotheses* 1994; 42: 323–327.
16. Reginster J Y, Deroisy R, Rovati L C, *et al.* Long-term effects of glucosamine sulphate on osteoarthritis progression: a randomised, placebo-controlled clinical trial. *Lancet* 2001; 357: 251–256.
17. Page J, Henry D. Consumption of NSAIDs and the development of congestive heart failure in elderly patients. *Arch Intern Med* 2000; 160: 777–784.
18. Lopes Vaz A. Double-blind clinical evaluation of the relative efficacy of ibuprofen and glucosamine sulphate in the management of osteoarthrosis of the knee in out-patients. *Curr Med Res Opin* 1982; 8: 145–149.
19. Setnikar I, Pacini A, Revel L. Antiarthritic effects of glucosamine sulphate studied in animal models. *Arzneim-Forsch/Drug Res* 1991; 41: 542–545.
20. Tapadinhas M J, Rivera I C, Bignamini A A. Oral glucosamine sulphate in the management of arthrosis. *Pharmatherapeutica* 1982; 3: 157–168.
21. Russell A L. Glucosamine in osteoarthritis and gastrointestinal disorders. *Med Hypoth* 1998; 51: 347–349.
22. Anderson G D. Glucosamine part III: dosing, safety and side-effects. *Dynamic Chiropract* 1998; 16: 28–30.
23. Adams M. Hype about glucosamine. *Lancet* 1999; 354: 353–354.
24. Altman R, Brandt K, Hochberg M, *et al.* Design and conduct of clinical trials of patients with osteoarthritis: recommendation from a task force of the Osteoarthritis Research Society. *Osteoarthritis Cartilage* 1996; 4: 217–243.

25. Quackwatch (1999). Glucosamine for arthritis. http://www.quackwatch.com/01 QuackeryRelated Topics/DSH/glucosamine.html (accessed 30 November 1999).
26. McAlindon T E, LaValley M P, Gulin J P, *et al.* Glucosamine and chondroitin for treatment of osteoarthritis – a systematic quality assessment and meta-analysis. *JAMA* 2000; 283: 1469–1475.
27. Towheed T E, Anastassiades T P. Glucosamine and chondroitin for treating symptoms of osteoarthritis – evidence is widely touted but incomplete. *JAMA* 2000; 283: 1483–1484.
28. Kayne S B, Wadeson K, MacAdam A. Is glucosamine an effective treatment for osteoarthritis? A meta-analysis. *Pharm J* 2000; 265: 759–763.
29. Eddington N D. Quality assurance of nutraceuticals in marketed products and raw materials: case study with chondroitin and glucosamine content in products and permeability across Caco-2 cells. Pharmacokinetics-Biopharmaceutics Laboratory, University of Maryland, Baltimore, MD, USA. Abstract Paper – Am Chem Soc 2000, 220th AGFD-149. CODEN:ACSRAL ISSN: 0065-7727. Journal; Meeting abstract written in English. AN 2000: 793181.
30. Adebowale A O, Liang Z, Eddington N D. Nutraceuticals, a call for quality control of delivery systems: a case study with chondroitin sulfate and glucosamine. *J Nutraceuticals Function Med Foods* 1999; 2: 15–30.
31. Houpt J B, McMillan R, Wein C, *et al.* Effect of glucosamine hydrochloride in the treatment of pain of osteoarthritis of the knee. *J Rheumatol* 1999; 26: 2423–2430.

# 3

# Octacosanol

Octacosanol, a compound found in the waxy outer layer of the leaves and fruit of many plants, is present in the normal diet in only very small amounts. To gain any health benefits, it must be taken as a supplement. Most studies assessing these benefits have been carried out using either a wheatgerm oil extract or policosanol, a natural mixture of primary alcohols purified from sugar cane (*Saccharum officinarum* L.) wax, the main component of which is octacosanol. There are many ways in which octacosanol has been used and these will be reviewed below.

## Properties and structure

Octacosanol is a 28-carbon chain aliphatic primary alcohol ($CH_3(CH_2)_{26}CH_2OH$) present in the superficial waxy layers of fruit, leaves and surface layer of many plants, as well as in whole grains. Its primary sources are the leaves of alfalfa and wheat and wheatgerm, but it is also obtained from various animal sources and is a component of paraffin.[1,2] Octacosanol was first isolated in the 1950s by Thomas Cureton.

## Uses of octacosanol

### Enhancement of athletic performance

It is well known that some athletes and sportsmen use various substances to help improve their performance. These 'ergogenic aids' include anabolic steroids, amphetamines and other substances that are now banned in sporting events. Most athletes now realise that as well as being illegal, many of these substances are harmful to health. This realisation means that they are turning to more natural products, including vitamins, protein mixtures, amino acids and other nutritional supplements. Because these substances are not licensed, very few have been researched fully, and as a result many claims made by manufacturers are unsubstantiated. Moreover, it is often difficult to assess the effectiveness of these products as any increased performance may also be due to improved training or diet.[3]

Octacosanol is a nutraceutical for which ergogenic claims have been made. Few scientific studies have been carried out to prove these claims and only a few papers have described trials using octacosanol in this way. Early experiments carried out by Cureton[4] claimed that after four to six weeks of octacosanol ingestion, there was an improvement in endurance activities, but these experiments have not been replicated.

More recently, a double-blind study using 16 students and lecturers of physical education measured grip and chest strength (as an indication of body strength), and reaction time to both auditory and visual stimuli after 1000 μg octacosanol was taken daily for eight weeks.[2] Results showed that reaction time to a visual stimulus and grip strength were improved, but that chest strength, endurance and reaction time in response to an auditory stimulus were unaffected. The authors concluded that although there were some benefits to supplementation with octacosanol, these did not appear to be as widespread as advertised. An experimental procedure carried out on mice, however, did show that octacosanol enhanced swimming endurance, possibly by converting lipids into energy, as in the test group there was also a significant decrease in liver triglycerides, serum triglycerides and total cholesterol.[5]

Another study in the 1980s used 33 male student athletes to test a combination of 29 nutritional supplements, including 2000 μg of octacosanol, developed by a team of scientists (Table 3.1).[6] Thirteen students consumed two of these packs daily and 20 students were used as controls. Diet and exercise regimens were unchanged during the eight-week study, however the diets of the subjects were not monitored. At the end of the supplemented period, all the test subjects showed a decrease in body fat, compared with only one in the control group, irrespective of initial levels. The supplemented subjects also showed a significant increase in muscle girth measurements, indicating the formation of lean body mass. This study was not a blind study and therefore placebo effects may have influenced the results. It was intended as a preliminary study to see if further investigations were warranted. Although the consistent results in the test group were impressive, since the packs contained many other supplements besides octacosanol, many of which are purported to enhance physical performance, no conclusions can be made without further studies on the isolated products.

**Table 3.1** Composition of the packs used to determine the effect of supplements on athletic performance

| | | |
|---|---|---|
| Tablet 1 | Vitamin $B_1$ | 25 mg |
| | Vitamin $B_2$ | 25 mg |
| | Vitamin $B_6$ | 25 mg |
| | Vitamin $B_{12}$ | 10 μg |
| | Pantothenic acid | 25 mg |
| | Folic acid | 400 μg |
| | Niacinamide | 25 mg |
| | Inositol | 25 mg |
| | Choline bitartrate | 25 mg |
| | L-Lysine HCl | 30 mg |
| | Vitamin C | 100 mg |
| | Neonatal bovine liver | 30 mg |
| | Pancrelipase | 50 mg |
| | Superoxide dismutase | 20 μg |
| | Catalase | 20 μg |
| | *Lactobacillus acidophilus* | 1 million |
| Tablet 2 | Orchic tissue | 40 mg |
| | Neonatal thymus tissue | 40 mg |
| | Neonatal spleen tissue | 40 mg |
| | Neonatal adrenal tissue | 20 mg |
| | Neonatal pituitary tissue | 20 mg |
| | Octacosanol | 2000 μg |
| | Gamma oryzanol | 5 mg |
| | Coenzyme Q10 | 50 μg |
| Tablet 3 | Chlorophyllin extract | 200 mg |
| | Vitamin C | 120 mg |
| Capsule 1 | L-Amino acid mixture | 500 mg |
| Capsule 2 | L-Arginine | 250 mg |
| | L-Ornithine | 250 mg |

From ref. 6.

## Motor neuron diseases

A small double-blind, controlled, randomised crossover study was carried out to determine the effects of octacosanol in patients with Parkinson's disease.[7] The 12-week trial involved ten patients with mild to moderate Parkinson's disease. One tablet of octacosanol 5 mg, or equivalent placebo, was taken for six weeks, three times a day with meals. Three patients improved significantly and another was himself able to identify the octacosanol period, although the results were not statistically significant. Side-effects were minimal and included position-related dizziness, worsening of carbidopa–levodopa-related dyskinesias and increased dystonic dyskinesia (causing one patient to discontinue the study). It is possible that these side-effects resulted from the high octacosanol dose used, as non-study patients reported improvements with 1 or 2 mg daily. The results indicate that some patients with mild Parkinson's disease symptoms are likely to benefit from this supplement. However, a much larger patient population is needed before clinically significant conclusions can be reached.

After these promising results with Parkinson's disease and encouraged by anecdotal reports of the benefit of octacosanol in amyotrophic lateral sclerosis (ALS), a controlled trial was carried out. ALS is a chronic degenerative motor neuron disease affecting the spinal cord and lower brainstem, and typically results in painless weakness and atrophy of the hands and spasticity and reflex hyperactivity of the legs. The disease is progressive, leading to death within three years in 50% of patients, but it can be prolonged and stabilise after some years of progression, and occasionally reverses.[8,9] A placebo-controlled, double-blind, crossover trial was carried out in which ALS patients received either 40 mg of active drug or placebo for three months and then the groups were crossed over.[10,11] Eleven out of 12 patients completed the trial. (In one patient there was unpredicted respiratory failure three weeks after the start of the study. He was hospitalised too far away from the medical centre and dropped out of the study. It was later found that he had received placebo.) The mean results showed no difference between octacosanol and placebo.

It can therefore be seen that to date, although anecdotal evidence seems to suggest otherwise, there is no clear indication for the use of octacosanol in motor neuron diseases such as Parkinson's disease or ALS.

### Lipid metabolism

Lipids are transported as lipoproteins in the blood. These include very low-density lipoprotein cholesterol (VLDL-C), low-density lipoprotein cholesterol (LDL-C) and high-density lipoprotein cholesterol (HDL-C). LDL-C is removed from the circulation by binding with both plasma membranes and HDL-C, and is a less concentrated form of cholesterol. An increased level of LDL-C (type II hypercholesterolaemia) can result from a deficiency in the binding mechanism; this may be due to a genetic defect (familial hypercholesterolaemia) or may be multifactorial due to genetics, diet and lifestyle. As well as primary hypercholesterolaemia, increased cholesterol levels may develop secondary to diabetes mellitus, hypothyroidism, pregnancy, renal failure, obesity, a high alcohol intake, poor diet and various drugs, such as beta-blockers, diuretics and oral contraceptives.[12,13]

Hypercholesterolaemia is known to be an important risk factor in the development of atherosclerosis and coronary heart disease (CHD) and studies have shown that a 1% decrease in serum cholesterol can lead to a 2% reduction in mortality. The aims of treatment are to increase HDL-C and decrease total cholesterol and LDL-C.[12,13]

Although diet can be used to lower cholesterol levels, in many cases this is insufficient and pharmacological intervention is required using lipid-lowering drugs, some of which cause side-effects. The statins, for example pravastatin and lovastatin, which are widely prescribed, have been reported to (rarely) cause hepatotoxicity, reflected by increases in serum transaminases, as well as myopathy leading to renal failure, reflected by increases in creatine phosphokinase.[14] The importance of these side-effects is augmented by the fact that statins are usually taken for a long period of time. Therefore the search for safe lipid-lowering agents continues, and the low incidence of side-effects makes octacosanol a promising choice.

### *Animal experimentation*

During motor endurance experiments on mice, it was noted that octacosanol caused altered hepatic and serum lipid concentrations, as stated above.[5] This led researchers to investigate the possible role of octacosanol and policosanol on serum lipids and its possible use as a cholesterol-lowering agent. Normocholesterolaemic animals have often been used in the evaluation of such agents. Since policosanol was shown to be a very safe substance, causing neither side-effects nor genetic changes in rodents and monkeys, much work has been carried out on the cholesterol-lowering effects of policosanol in these animals.[15]

In one study,[15] three groups of seven rabbits received 5, 50 and 200 mg/kg of policosanol and a control group of ten animals received placebo. The normal cholesterol diet was similar in all groups, as was weight gain during the study. Blood samples were taken before and after the four weeks of treatment. Cholesterol, triglycerides, HDL-C, and LDL-C were all evaluated. All doses significantly reduced total cholesterol and LDL-C in a dose-dependent way, whilst HDL-C was unchanged. This indicates that the cholesterol-lowering effects of policosanol on normocholesterolaemic subjects is due to a decrease in

LDL-C, which could be due to the degradation of this lipoprotein. Lipid-lowering drugs must not only reduce cholesterol, but also the specific lipoproteins that are known to be a risk factor in atherogenic disease. Since high LDL-C levels are one such risk, policosanol could have a place as a hypolipidaemic drug, based on these preliminary findings.

Another animal study on the effect of octacosanol used rats as the experimental model. In this study, both rats on a normal diet and those fed a high-fat diet were used in a three-part experimental procedure.[1] One experiment looked at the effect of supplementation with octacosanol on four groups of six rats. A significant decrease in the weight of perirenal adipose tissue was found, without a significant difference in body weight. Two further experiments examined the effect of octacosanol on the enzymes involved in lipid metabolism and on the rate of total fatty acid oxidation in two groups of ten rats. The activities of the enzymes were affected by the fat content of the diet, but octacosanol had no effect. However, the rate-limiting step in the esterification of fatty acid into triacylglycerol was decreased by octacosanol, suggesting that a step in the biosynthesis of cholesterol had been inhibited. In the rats fed a normal diet these changes were not seen, indicating that the octacosanol effect may depend on the dietary fat content.

### Human trials

The first cholesterol-lowering effects of policosanol in human subjects were recorded in 1992.[16] Previously, doses of up to 1000 mg policosanol had been given to human volunteers with no significant side-effects and therefore it was assumed that it was safe to use human subjects to test the lipid effects of policosanol. A double-blind study was carried out in 38 healthy volunteers, with normal cholesterol values, on a normal diet. They were given placebo, 10 mg or 20 mg policosanol daily (as 5 mg twice daily or 10 mg twice daily). After four weeks, those in the 10-mg dose group showed significantly decreased serum cholesterol, but LDL-C and HDL-C were unchanged. At a dose of 20 mg policosanol daily, there were significant reductions in both cholesterol and LDL-C, whilst HDL-C values were increased. In the placebo group there was an opposite trend, possibly due to changes in diet, which was not monitored during the study. In these healthy subjects, policosanol was well tolerated and safe, as well as effective in lowering serum cholesterol and LDL-C in a dose-dependent way.

In another study,[17] 26 elderly patients with primary hypercholesterolaemia received placebo, 1 mg policosanol, or 10 mg policosanol every evening for 24 weeks. Again there were promising results and serum total cholesterol was significantly reduced in a dose-dependent fashion, suggesting that policosanol is an effective drug for elderly, hypercholesterolaemic patients. There were no adverse reactions, and biochemical and clinical findings were unchanged. This demonstrated that policosanol is a safe supplement even for a relatively long duration of treatment.

To test the effect of successive doses of policosanol on the lipid profile and tolerability of treatment, a double-blind study was carried out on 33 outpatients with primary hypercholesterolaemia.[18] To obtain a baseline reading the patients were put on a low-fat diet for four weeks and all lipid-lowering medication was stopped. At this stage a lipid profile was taken from blood samples. The double-blind trial then commenced and for six weeks the subjects received two policosanol 5 mg tablets daily (10 mg daily) or placebo, and then for a further six weeks they took two tablets twice daily (20 mg daily) or placebo. Treatment with the lower dose showed a significant reduction in total cholesterol and LDL-C by 16.8% and 22% respectively, but in the placebo group changes were insignificant. The higher dose further reduced these levels by 20.5% and 29.1% respectively. Although triglyceride and VLDL-C values were unchanged, HDL-C values were increased in both parts of the trial, whilst values in the placebo group decreased. Two patients in the policosanol group and five in the placebo group reported mild side-effects. This trial again indicates that policosanol is a useful and safe lipid-lowering supplement.

### *Patients with type II hypercholesterolaemia*

Many trials have been carried out using policosanol in patients with type II hypercholesterolaemia.[12,19–24] A summary is shown in Table 3.2.

In the randomised, double-blind, placebo-controlled studies, a baseline lipid profile was taken after a period of time on a low-fat diet, during which all lipid-lowering medication was discontinued. In all cases, policosanol was shown to significantly reduce both total cholesterol and LDL-C. Triglyceride values were unchanged in all but one experiment, in which values were reduced, and changes in HDL-C were either not significant or increased in all trials. In the study by Castano *et al.*,[23] the patients selected were also suffering from hypertension and many were receiving antihypertensive medications such as beta-blockers and diuretics. These drugs could affect the lipid profile, and this may explain why the reduction in values in this trial was less than in the other

**Table 3.2** Several trials using policosanol in patients with type II hypercholesterolaemia, showing values compared with the baseline and/or placebo

| *Ref* | *Length of study* | *Dose* | *Patient number* | *Total cholesterol* | *LDL-C* | *HDL-C* | *Triglycerides* |
|---|---|---|---|---|---|---|---|
| 19 | 12 months | 5 mg o.d. | 52 | ⇓15.3% | ⇓23.7% | ⇔ | ⇔ |
| 20 | 6 weeks | 5 mg b.d. | 45 | ⇓16.2% | ⇓21.5% | ⇔ | ⇔ |
| 21 | 12 months | 5 mg b.d. | 74 | ⇓17.2% | ⇓26.4% | ⇑13.5% | ⇔ |
| 22 | 12 months | 5 mg b.d. | 62 | ⇓15.6% | ⇓23.1% | ⇔ | ⇔ |
| 23 | 12 months | 5 mg b.d. | 58 | ⇓13% | ⇓19.1% | ⇑17.1% | ⇔ |
| 24 | 12 weeks | 5 mg o.d.[a] | 437 | ⇓13%[b] | ⇓18.2%[b] | ⇑15.5%[b] | ⇔ |
| | 12 weeks | 10 mg o.d | | ⇓17.4% | ⇓25.6% | ⇑28.4% | ⇓5.2% |
| 12 | 12 weeks | 5 mg o.d.[a] | 244 | ⇓12.6%[b] | ⇓17.7%[b] | ⇑16.5%[b] | ⇔ |
| | 12 weeks | 10 mg o.d. | | ⇓16.8% | ⇓25.4% | ⇑29.3% | ⇔ |

o.d., once daily; b.d., twice daily; ⇓ significant decrease; ⇑ significant increase; ⇔ no significant change.

[a]5 mg daily were taken for 12 weeks followed by 10 mg daily for 12 weeks.

[b]First result after 12 weeks; second result after 24 weeks.

trials. In the trial by Mas *et al.*,[24] patients had at least two other coronary risk factors such as obesity, hypertension and diabetes and were taking medication for these conditions. Even in these patients, there were no significant side-effects, nor were there any interactions between policosanol and other medication being used.

Castano *et al.*[12] studied the effect of policosanol in postmenopausal women. After the menopause, women have higher levels of serum total cholesterol and LDL-C than men of the same age do. LDL-C levels have been shown to rise and therefore postmenopausal women are at greater risk from CHD, due to reduced serum oestrogen, which has anti-atherogenic effects. This study involved women who were not receiving hormone replacement therapy (HRT), which has been shown to reduce the risk for CHD by the effect of oestrogen on lipid levels. Policosanol was well tolerated in this population, with only a few mild adverse effects and one subject complaining of moderate gastrointestinal effects in the test group (although there were several serious adverse effects in the placebo group). The results show that policosanol is an effective cholesterol-lowering agent in postmenopausal women.

A randomised, double-blind study was carried out to compare the effects of 10 mg/day policosanol and 10 mg/day pravastatin in older type II hypercholesterolaemia patients with coronary risk, over eight weeks.[25] Policosanol was more effective in reducing LDL-C levels, the ratio of LDL-C to HDL-C, and the ratio of total cholesterol to HDL-C. Policosanol was also more effective in inhibiting platelet aggregation. Although both treatments were safe and well tolerated, pravastatin induced moderate but significant increases in serum transaminase. The authors concluded that policosanol 10 mg/day was a better choice of cholesterol-lowering therapy than pravastatin 10 mg/day, for elderly type II hypercholesterolaemia patients with coronary risk.

### *Non-insulin-dependent diabetes mellitus patients*

In non-insulin-dependent diabetes mellitus (NIDDM), hyperglycaemia may induce atherosclerosis leading to coronary heart disease, which is a main cause of death in these patients. It is therefore important to maintain low cholesterol levels in NIDDM patients by using glycaemic control, dietary measures and medication. Policosanol was used in a double-blind study of these patients.[26] Thirty-two patients with stable glycaemic control were given policosanol 5 mg twice a day for 12 weeks, or a placebo. Both cholesterol and LDL-C were significantly reduced in the test group and showed a non-significant upward trend in the placebo group. Side-effects were mild, and at week 12 no side-effects were reported in the policosanol group and the treatment did not affect glycaemic control. This study shows the possible place of policosanol as a cholesterol-lowering drug in patients with controlled NIDDM.

Another study was carried out to compare 10 mg/day policosanol and 20 mg/day lovastatin in patients with hypercholesterolaemia and NIDDM.[27] In this randomised, double-blind study, 53 patients received either policosanol or lovastatin daily for 12 weeks. Both treatments were effective in lowering LDL-C and total cholesterol, without affecting glucose control. Policosanol was found to be safe and well tolerated, whereas lovastatin caused increased serum values of aspartate aminotransferase, creatine phosphokinase and alkaline phosphatase, as well as causing more frequent adverse effects (including five patients who withdrew from the study).

## Inhibition of thromboxane production

### *Platelet aggregation*

Trauma to blood cells can lead to the activation of the clotting cascade, which results in platelet activation and aggregation. These aggregates form a plug, which can cause cerebral ischaemia and thrombosis. Thromboxane $A_2$ ($TXA_2$), a cyclooxygenase metabolite found in platelets, can initiate aggregation and is involved in the physiology of experimental myocardial ischaemia and in human heart disease. $TXA_2$ is converted to thromboxane $B_2$ ($TXB_2$), a more stable and less active metabolite, which is therefore often used as a measurement of *in vivo* platelet aggregation.[13]

As high cholesterol levels are a major risk factor for coronary artery disease and platelet function is an important factor in occlusive vascular arterial disease, a drug with both cholesterol-lowering and antiplatelet effects is of interest. Inhibition of platelet adhesion and aggregation should reduce thrombus formation and therefore prevent the development of atherosclerosis.[28,29] Since some lipid-lowering drugs also have an effect on platelet aggregation, this possibility was investigated for policosanol in a series of animal experiments.[30] Groups of ten rats were used in a controlled study which found that policosanol at doses of 5–20 mg/kg, had an anti-aggregation effect on platelets when compared with placebo. The mechanism was believed to be related to inhibition of arachidonic acid metabolism, as a subsequent dose of 25 mg/kg inhibited $TXA_2$ in the rat clotted whole blood.

In another experiment, policosanol at a higher dose of 25–200 mg/kg was used to treat adult Mongolian gerbils before ligation of the common carotid artery, which usually leads to approximately 90% of the animals dying due to cerebral infarction.[31] In the policosanol-treated gerbils, there were significantly lower levels of $TXB_2$ than in controls, indicating that there was less platelet aggregation. A dose–effect relationship for $TXB_2$ was seen up to a dose of 50 mg/kg, at which point the effect was maximal. However, significantly reduced mortality from cerebral infarction was observed in gerbils that received 200 mg/kg (but not at the lower doses), despite this being far above the maximum dose.

In a second part of this experiment, the synergistic effect of co-administering policosanol and aspirin was investigated. Aspirin is the drug most commonly used for cerebral ischaemia and thrombosis and is a cyclooxygenase inhibitor that inhibits the formation of $TXA_2$. The results showed that this combination significantly protected the experimental animals, even when policosanol was given at the lower dose of 25 mg/kg. Both of these animal studies indicate the involvement of policosanol in prostaglandin and thromboxane pathways.

A number of human studies have also been carried out. The effect of doses of 5–50 mg policosanol was investigated using 87 healthy human volunteers in a randomised, placebo-controlled, double-blind study.[32] Both single-dose and repeated doses were used. Blood samples were withdrawn before and two hours after the policosanol or placebo dose, and the aggregating agents adenosine diphosphate (ADP), adrenaline (epinephrine) and collagen were added. In the single-dose study, platelet aggregation in response to ADP and adrenaline was significantly decreased, with doses of 10, 25 and 50 mg policosanol, compared with the placebo group, but responses to collagen were not altered. When policosanol was given at a dose of 20 mg daily for seven days, platelet aggregation was again significantly decreased, and although there was a decrease in the collagen-treated blood samples, this was not significant. Significant doses were from 10 mg daily, but the lower dose of 5 mg had no effect. The authors suggested that the increased reaction to ADP and adrenaline rather than to collagen implied that policosanol affected the fibrinogen-binding site on platelets. Higher doses and longer duration could lead to better antiplatelet effects.

When policosanol and aspirin were compared in a study using 43 healthy volunteers, it was found that 20 mg daily of policosanol was as effective as 100 mg daily of aspirin in reducing induced platelet aggregation. Combination therapy (100 mg aspirin plus 20 mg policosanol) showed advantages over individual therapy.[33]

The effects of policosanol (10 mg daily) on blood aggregation were also determined in a four-week, double-blind, placebo-controlled study using 27 type II hypercholesterolaemic patients.[29] There was a significant decrease in aggregation caused by both arachidonic acid and collagen. Hypercholesterolaemic patients are often hypersensitive to platelet-inducing agents, and therefore policosanol could be a promising supplement for these patients, both lowering cholesterol levels and reducing platelet effects.

Another placebo-controlled, double-blind trial was carried out using patients with intermittent claudication.[28] This is an occlusive peripheral arterial disease, characterised by the inability of the patient to walk a distance without pain and a feeling of coldness in the lower limbs. Walking distance for inclusion into the trial was between 50 and 300 m as measured on a treadmill (no pain at 50 m, pain beginning before 300 m). Sixty two outpatients were randomised to receive test or placebo for six months. Ten of these dropped out before the end of the trial; six (who were all in the placebo group) from side-effects and the others for personal reasons. The test group received 10 mg policosanol twice daily, and all other medication was allowed, except for drugs acting specifically on platelet aggregation, such as aspirin and dipyridamole. The results showed a significant improvement in walking distance of over 60% in the test group, compared with the controls, where distances remained stable. Moreover, far more adverse effects were reported in the placebo group, including seven that were serious and most of which were vascular. There were three minor and transient side-effects reported in the policosanol group.

These results are very promising; as well as demonstrating its positive effects on patients with intermittent claudication, they also reinforce the good tolerability of policosanol.

### *Myocardial infarction*

Since policosanol is known to reduce platelet aggregation and $TXB_2$, an experimental animal study was carried out using 48 rats to determine the effect of oral pre-treatment with policosanol 2 hours before isoprenaline-induced myocardial infarction. Policosanol reduced the size of the myocardial injury and also decreased the number of polymorphonuclear neutrophils (PMNs) and mast cells in the damaged areas. These cells play an important role in cardiac cell damage, so a reduction in their numbers indicates less damage. The authors concluded that more work is necessary to determine the clinical value of their findings.[34]

### Treatment of gastric ulcers

D-002, a natural mixture of higher primary alcohols isolated from beeswax and containing 17.49% octacosanol, was investigated for its anti-ulcer activity.[35] Ten rats were treated with 5, 25 or 50 mg/kg D-002 or 25 mg/kg cimetidine. One hour later, ulceration was induced with either indometacin or 60% ethanol, and then the rats were killed and examined for ulceration. D-002 showed similar results to cimetidine in significantly preventing both indometacin-induced and ethanol-induced ulcers. One of the main factors in the formation of these ulcers is the presence of gastric acid, but in a further experiment, D-002 was shown to be independent of gastric acid. The possible role of D-002 as a cytoprotective agent where the mechanism is not dependent on gastric acid was further investigated.[36] The results suggest the possible role of prostaglandins in the gastroprotective effects of D-002, rather than the inhibition of gastric acid as in the case of cimetidine.

## Conclusions

Clinical trials have shown that octacosanol (policosanol) is a useful supplement in certain circumstances, however many claims, such as those for improving athletes' performances, have yet to be proved. The main effects have been seen in the area of lipid metabolism and cholesterol lowering, as well as platelet function. With continued study in this field it may be that octacosanol will turn out to be a useful supplement in gastric ulceration and motor neuron disease, but as yet it is too early to predict. Octacosanol was well tolerated and no significant side-effects were reported in any of the studies, even when it was taken at a dose of 40 mg daily.[10] There seems good reason, therefore, to continue researching the usefulness of this nutraceutical.

## References

1. Kato S, Karino K, Hasegawa J, *et al.* Octacosanol affects lipid metabolism in rats fed on a high fat diet. *Br J Nutr* 1995; 73: 433–442.
2. Saint-John M, McNaughton L. Octacosanol ingestion and its effects on metabolic responses to submaximal cycle ergometry, reaction time and chest and grip strength. *Int Clin Nutr Rev* 1986; 6: 81–87.
3. Beltz S D, Doering P L. Efficacy of nutritional supplements used by athletes. *Clin Pharm* 1993; 12: 900–908.
4. Cureton T K. *The Physiological Effects of Wheat Germ Oil on Humans in Exercise.* Chicago: Charles C Thomas, 1972.

5. Shimura S, Hasegawa T, Takano S, *et al.* Studies on the effect of octacosanol on motor endurance in mice. *Nutr Rep Int* 1987; 36: 1029–1038.
6. Cockerill D L, Bucci L R. Increases in muscle girth and decreases in body fat associated with a nutritional supplement program. *Chiro Sports Med* 1987; 1: 73–76.
7. Snider S R. Octacosanol in Parkinsonism. *Ann Neurol* 1984; 16: 723.
8. Andreoli T E, Bennett J C, Carpenter C C J, *et al. Cecil Essentials of Medicine*, 4th edn. Pennsylvania: W B Saunders, 1997.
9. Tandan R, Bradley W G. Amyotrophic lateral sclerosis, pt.1 *Ann Neurol* 1985; 18: 271–280.
10. Norris F H, Denys E H, Fallat R J. Trial of octacosanol on amyotrophic lateral sclerosis. *Neurology* 1986; 36: 1263–1264.
11. Norris F H, Denys E H. Nutritional supplements in amyotrophic lateral sclerosis. *Adv Exp Med Biol* 1987; 209: 183–189.
12. Castano G, Mas R, Fernandez L, *et al.* Effects of policosanol on postmenopausal women with type II hypercholesterolemia. *Gynecol Endocrinol* 2000; 14: 187–195.
13. Craig C R, Stitzel R E. *Modern Pharmacology*, 4th edn. Boston: Little, Browne Company 1994.
14. Farnier M, Davignon J. Current and future treatment of hyperlipidemia: the role of statins. *Am J Cardiol* 1998; 82: 3J–10J.
15. Arruzazabala M L, Carbajal D, Mas R, *et al.* Cholesterol-lowering effects of policosanol in rabbits. *Biol Res* 1994; 27: 205–208.
16. Hernandez F, Illnait J, Mas R, *et al.* Effect of policosanol on serum lipids and lipoproteins in healthy volunteers. *Curr Ther Res* 1992; 51: 568–575.
17. Pons P, Jimenez A, Rodrigues M, *et al.* Effects of policosanol in elderly hypercholesterolemic patients. *Curr Ther Res* 1993; 53: 265–269.
18. Aneiros E, Calderon B, Mas R, *et al.* Effect of successive dose increases of policosanol on the lipid profile and tolerability of treatment. *Curr Ther Res* 1993; 54: 304–312.
19. Pons P, Rodriguez M, Mas R, *et al.* One-year efficacy and safety of policosanol in patients with type II hypercholesterolaemia. *Curr Ther Res* 1994; 55: 1084–1092.
20. Aneiros E, Mas R, Calderon B, *et al.* Effect of policosanol in lowering cholesterol levels in patients with type II hypercholesterolaemia. *Curr Ther Res* 1995: 56: 176–182.
21. Castano G, Mas R, Nodarse M, *et al.* One year study of the efficacy and safety of policosanol (5mg twice daily) in the treatment of type II hypercholesterolaemia. *Curr Ther Res* 1995; 56: 296–304.
22. Castano G, Canetti M, Moreira M, *et al.* Efficacy and tolerability of policosanol in elderly patients with type II hypercholesterolaemia: a 12-month study. *Curr Ther Res* 1995; 56: 819–823.
23. Castano G, Tula L, Canetti M, *et al.* Effects of policosanol in hypertensive patients with type II hypercholesterolaemia. *Curr Ther Res* 1996; 57: 691–698.
24. Mas R, Castano G, Illnait J, *et al.* Effects of policosanol in patients with type II hypercholesterolaemia and additional coronary risk factors. *Clin Pharmacol Ther* 1999; 65: 439–447.
25. Castano G, Mas R, Arruzazabala M L, *et al.* Effects of policosanol and

pravastatin on lipid profile, platelet aggregation and endothelemia in older hypercholesterolemic patients. *Int J Clin Pharmacol Res* 1999; 19: 105–116.
26. Torres O, Agramonte A J, Illnait J, *et al.* Treatment of hypercholesterolemia in NIDDM with policosanol. *Diabetes Care* 1995; 18: 393–397.
27. Crespo N, Illnait J, Mas R, *et al.* Comparative study of the efficacy and tolerability of policosanol and lovastatin in patients with hypercholesterolemia and noninsulin dependent diabetes mellitus. *Int J Clin Pharmacol Res* 1999; 19: 117–127.
28. Castano G, Mas R, Roca J, *et al.* A double-blind, placebo-controlled study of the effects of policosanol in patients with intermittent claudication. *Angiology* 1999; 50: 123–130.
29. Arruzazabala M L, Mas R, Molina V, *et al.* Effects of policosanol on platelet aggregation in type II hypercholesterolaemic patients. *Tissue Reactions* 1998; 20: 119–124.
30. Arruzazabala M L, Carbajal D, Mas R, *et al.* Effects of policosanol on platelet aggregation in rats. *Thromb Res* 1993; 69: 321–332.
31. Arruzazabala M L, Molina V, Carbajal D, *et al.* Effect of policosanol on cerebral ischemia in mongolian gerbils. *Prostaglandins Leukot Essent Fatty Acids* 1993; 49: 695–696.
32. Valdes S, Arruzazabala M L, Fernandez L, *et al.* Effect of policosanol on platelet aggregation in healthy volunteers. *Int J Clin Pharmacol Res* 1996; 16: 67–72.
33. Arruzazabala M L, Valdes S, Mas R, *et al.* Comparative study of policosanol, aspirin and the combination therapy policosanol-aspirin on platelet aggregation in healthy volunteers. *Pharmacol Res* 1997; 36: 293 abstract.
34. Noa M, Herrera M, Magraner J, *et al.* Effect of policosanol on isoprenaline-induced myocardial necrosis in rats. *J Pharm Pharmacol* 1994; 46: 282–285.
35. Carbajal D, Molina V, Valdes S, *et al.* Anti-ulcer activity of higher primary alcohols of beeswax. *J Pharm Pharmacol* 1995; 47: 731–733.
36. Carbajal D, Molina V, Valdes S, *et al.* Possible cytoprotective mechanism in rats of D-002, an anti-ulcerogenic product isolated from beeswax. *J Pharm Pharmacol* 1996; 48: 858–860.

# 4

# Proanthocyanidins and grape products

The proanthocyanidins (PACs) are a group of phytochemicals that have been attracting much attention both among the general public and among health professionals. A subgroup of the bioflavonoids (once called vitamin P), PACs occur naturally in many fruits, vegetables, nuts and seeds, as well as in the flowers, roots and bark of many plants.[1] It is well known that the ingestion of a diet high in fruits and vegetables offers protection against a variety of diseases, resulting in the generally recommended 'five a day' diet, which encourages people to eat at least five portions of fruits and vegetables each day. It is thought that this protection results from the increase of antioxidants in the body. In a number of studies the preparation known as grape seed proanthocyanidin extract (GSPE) has been shown to prevent the development of certain disease states and it seems that it exerts these effects by acting as an antioxidant.

## Properties and structure

Also known as vegetable tannins, polyphenols or condensed tannins, because of their early use in the tanning of leathers, PACs are found in the leaves, fruits, bark, seeds and roots of many plants. Rich dietary sources include fruits such as apples (*Malus*), grapes (*Vitis vinifera*), blackberries and raspberries (*Rubus*), bilberries and cranberries (*Vaccinium*), rosehips (*Rosa*) and hawthorn (*Crataegus*)[2] and PACs have been used in foods, livestock feeds, beverages (such as wine and tea) and herbal preparations for many years. PACs are the main precursors of the blue-violet and red colouring in plants.[3]

The properties of the PACs or polyphenols have been studied and described.[4] In the natural state, polyphenol–polyphenol interactions ensure minimum solubility in aqueous media. Molecular weights vary from 500 to 4000 and reactions include complexation reactions with metal ions, complex formation with proteins and polysaccharides and antioxidation reactions.

The polyphenol structure is based on the flavan-3-ol unit, which can be either *trans* (catechin) or *cis* (epicatechin) (Figure 4.1). As the

(a) 2,3 *trans*(+)-catechin

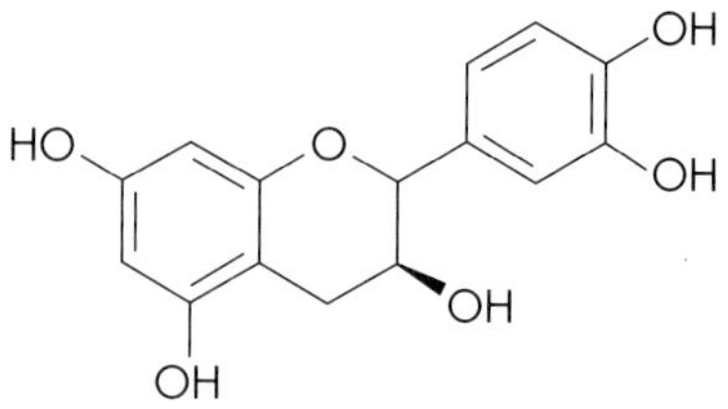

(b) 2,3 *cis*(–)-epicatechin

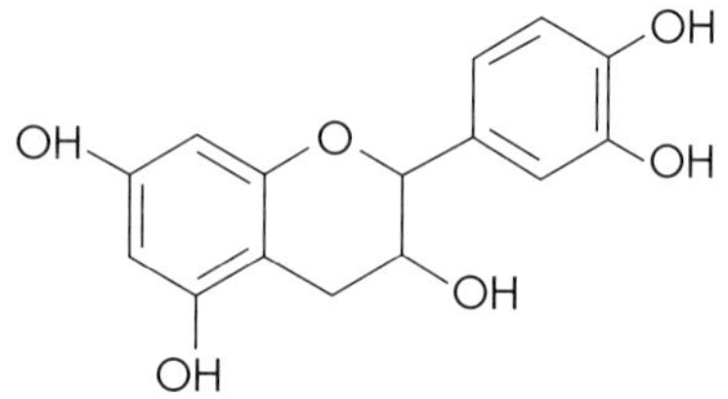

(c) Dimer B1

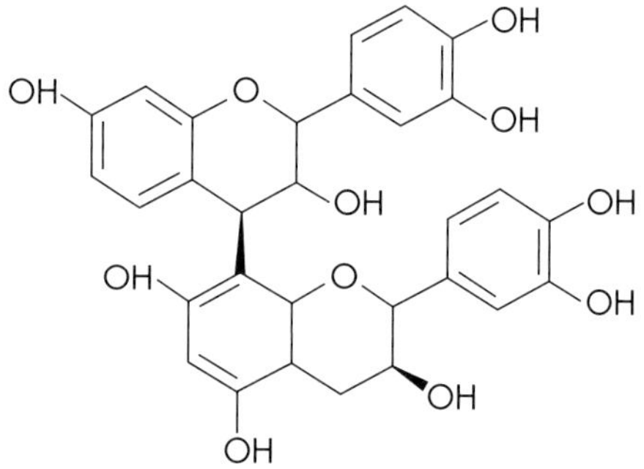

**Figure 4.1** Basic structures of the proanthocyanidins:[4,7,8] (a) 2,3 *trans*(+)-catechin, (b) 2,3 *cis*(−)-epicatechin and (c) dimer B1, a dimeric proanthocyanidin that occurs in grapes and cranberries.

monomers join together to form dimers, trimers and other oligomers, many different structures are formed due to changes in stereochemistry. Usually there are five to seven aromatic rings with 12–16 phenolic groups. Dimeric proanthocyanidins have also been called proanthocyanidin B1, B2, B3 and B4 depending on the configuration of catechin and epicatechin subunits, and they are classified according to the hydroxylation of rings 1 and 3. The dimeric proanthocyanidin B1 is also called epicatechin-(4b-8)-catechin and is found in grapes and cranberries.[2–8]

PACs were first extracted from pine bark in 1951 and from grape seeds in 1970.[3] Extraction from the plant material is based on their preferential solubilities in organic solvents; usually 80% methanol,

ethanol or acetone is used for the water-soluble oligomers that have two to six units. The aqueous extract is then partitioned with an organic solvent, such as ethyl acetate. Both thin-layer chromatography (TLC) and column absorption chromatography are used to separate out the different components. The intense colours seen with ultraviolet light can then detect the different fractions.[9] High-performance liquid chromatography (HPLC) and mass spectrometry (MS) are also employed.

## Uses of proanthocyanidins

### As antioxidants

Oxidation is a process that occurs naturally in the body when oxygen combines with reduced carbon-based molecules (carbohydrates or fats) and produces energy. This normal process propagates short-lived intermediates, known as free radicals. These are molecules with one or more unpaired electrons, and as such they are highly reactive. Some free radicals escape and initiate further oxidation, setting up a chain reaction. Since free radicals are difficult to measure directly, the molecular damage they cause is measured instead. Although free radicals will react with any type of molecule, the most frequent damage is caused to carbohydrates, lipids, nucleic acids and proteins. This is known as oxidative stress.[10–12]

Oxidative stress is the general phenomenon of oxidant exposure and antioxidant depletion, or increased oxidant–antioxidant balance. The ideal situation for proper metabolic function is to provide enough pro-oxidants (food) for the generation of sufficient but not excess energy, so that not too many free radicals are released. Antioxidants, or free radical scavengers, are the molecular defences that prevent these free radicals from causing excess cellular damage. Natural (unrefined) foods contain antioxidants but in processing many of these are lost. In addition, environmental pollutants, radiation, pesticides, medications, spicy or deep-fried foods, direct and second-hand cigarette smoke, as well as physical stress can produce free radicals. These cause degeneration of body tissues from oxidative stress, leading to disease states.[13,14]

Many diseases are thought to be the result of free radical reactions that occur in human metabolism in the absence of free radical scavengers. Indeed, the products of oxidation reactions can cause much damage, including loss of function from direct oxidation, such as the oxidation of membrane lipids leading to altered membrane permeability, or loss of enzyme regulation or activity from the oxidation of proteins. Moreover, products of oxidation can result in inappropriate cell responses.[10] Therefore, the ingestion of certain antioxidant nutrients may be of use to prevent the damage caused by these processes. Examples of potent antioxidants include vitamin C, vitamin E, betacarotene, zinc, selenium and antioxidant enzymes such as glutathione, superoxide dismutase and catalase.[14] Moreover, many everyday foods are potent antioxidants. Table 4.1 shows the serving equivalents of the antioxidant activity in a variety of foods and drinks, based on polyphenol content.[15]

This free radical theory is associated with a long list of diseases that includes cancer, autoimmune disease, cardiovascular disease, trauma, gastrointestinal problems, cataract, Alzheimer's disease, psoriasis, stroke and AIDS. The wide range of diseases suggests that tissue and cellular injury caused by free radical damage could indeed be the reason for most human illness.[10,16,17]

For a PAC to be classed as an antioxidant it must be able to delay, slow or prevent oxidative damage when in low concentration relative to the substrate to be oxidised. The availability of the phenolic hydrogens of the PACs to be donated predicts the antioxidant characteristics. Also, the resulting product must be stable on further oxidation. Several PACs have been shown to be good antioxidants, including an extract from hawthorn (*Crataegus monogyna*),[18] which has long been used in herbal medicine.

Most of the pharmacological uses of PACs are related to their antioxidant properties. In particular, grape seed extract has been shown to be a potent antioxidant. A study was carried out to assess the antioxidant strength of a grape seed proanthocyanidin extract (GSPE) by comparing the concentration–response of the free radical scavenging ability (antioxidation) with that of vitamin C and vitamin E succinate

**Table 4.1** The equivalent antioxidant activities of different foods

| *Food* | *Serving size* |
|---|---|
| Red wine | 1 glass (150 ml) |
| White wine | 12 glasses |
| Tea | 2 cups |
| Apples | 5 fruits |
| Blackcurrant juice | 3.5 glasses |
| Beer | 500 ml |
| Orange juice | 7 glasses |
| Apple juice | 20 glasses |

(VES).[1] In this *in vitro* experiment, oxygen free radicals including superoxide anion and hydroxyl radicals were generated and then measured. Chemiluminescence, a general assay for the production of reactive species, and chemical assay with cytochrome *c*, which is specific for superoxide anion production, were used to observe the inhibition of these free radicals by the antioxidants. Results showed a very good concentration-dependent response for GSPE in the inhibition of superoxide anion and hydroxyl radical production, with similar results obtained when inhibition of superoxide production was measured by the cytochrome *c* method (A) and by chemiluminescence (B), as shown in Table 4.2. Vitamin C and VES also showed free radical scavenging properties but GSPE was a better antioxidant.

A similar study was carried out *in vivo* to compare the antioxidant properties of GSPE, vitamin C, VES and betacarotene.[13,16] GSPE (25–100 mg/kg) dissolved in water, vitamin C (100 mg/kg) dissolved in water, VES (100 mg/kg) dissolved in corn oil and betacarotene (50 mg/kg) dissolved in corn oil were fed using a feeding needle to groups of four mice each morning for seven days. Lipid peroxidation (oxidative stress) was induced by 12-O-tetradecanoylphorbol-13-acetate (TPA) on the eighth day, 2 hours after the injection. Two hours later, the mice were killed and hepatic and brain tissues were removed. Results were obtained for reactive oxygen species production by measuring chemiluminescence and assay with cytochrome *c*, superoxide anion production by chemical assay, lipid peroxidation by absorbance, and DNA fragmentation by centrifugation followed by absorbance (Table 4.3).

It can be seen that GSPE provided the best protection in all categories at the doses used. (It was interesting to note that a combination

**Table 4.2** The percentage inhibition of free radicals by grape seed proanthocyanidin extract (GSPE)[1]

| *GSPE (mg/L)* | *A – % inhibition of superoxide anion production (cytochrome c)* | *B – % inhibition of superoxide anion production (chemiluminescence)* | *C – % inhibition of hydroxyl radical production (chemiluminescence)* |
|---|---|---|---|
| 5 | 17 | 19 | 18 |
| 25 | 59 | 62 | 60 |
| 50 | 72 | 76 | 70 |
| 100 | 81 | 79 | 78 |
| 200 | 89 | 88 | 90 |

**Table 4.3** The percentage inhibition of 12-*O*-tetradecanoylphorbol-13-acetate (TPA)-induced reactive oxygen species with various antioxidants[13,16]

| | *Decrease in TPA-induced free radical production (%)* | *Decrease in TPA-induced DNA fragmentation (liver) (%)* | *Decrease in TPA-induced DNA fragmentation (brain) (%)* |
|---|---|---|---|
| GSPE | 70 | 47 | 50 |
| Vitamin E succinate (VES) | 40 | 30 | 31 |
| Vitamin C | 16 | 10 | 14 |
| VES plus vitamin C | 48 | 38 | 40 |
| Betacarotene | 17 | 11 | 11 |

of vitamin C and VES provided better protection than the individual vitamins alone.) These results suggest that GSPE is not only an efficient antioxidant *in vitro*, but also *in vivo*, where it is absorbed and distributed in target organs, such as the liver and brain, and as such it may be useful in preventing tissue damage by oxidation.

GSPE has also been shown to offer protection against smokeless tobacco-induced oxidative damage in a culture of human oral keratinocytes.[14] Pre-treatment of tobacco-treated cells with 100 mg/ml GSPE resulted in a reduction of cell death of approximately 85%.

## Atherosclerosis

Cholesterol is found in the bloodstream with triglycerides, phospholipids and proteins in carrier plasma lipoproteins. Low-density lipoprotein cholesterol (LDL-C) carries cholesterol from foods and the liver to the cells and is thought of as 'bad' cholesterol, whereas high-density lipoprotein cholesterol (HDL-C) carries cholesterol from the cells back to the liver where it is converted to bile ready for excretion and is thought of as 'good' cholesterol. For many years cholesterol has been thought to be the cause of the rising deaths from cardiovascular disease (CVD) and atherosclerosis. It seems that if levels of LDL-C accumulate because of the ingestion of high levels of saturated fat, the excess cholesterol is deposited in the arteries, increasing the risk of CVD.[11]

*The benefits of red wine – the French paradox*

In 1989 the World Health Organization conducted a worldwide study to establish the mortality rates from CVD in different populations. It was found that although risk factors such as dietary intake of saturated fats, blood pressure, obesity and serum cholesterol values in France were similar to those in other western countries such as Britain and the USA, deaths from CVD were much lower. This phenomenon became known as the 'French paradox'.[19] It was found that these differences in mortality were due to the high intake of red wine in France. Moderate intake of red wine at levels of about 20–30 g per day was shown to reduce the risk of death from CVD by as much as 40%. When the CVD risk in Toulouse, France was compared with those in Belfast and Glasgow the difference was even greater. Because consumption of wine in these areas is low, but the consumption of alcoholic drinks overall is comparable, it was concluded that it was the red wine and not alcohol or spirits that led to this finding.[20,21]

Wine is a fermentation product of the juice (or must) of grapes. The fermentation process produces many chemical changes, and wine is a unique product, rather than just grape juice with alcohol added. Different wines vary according to the starter grapes used and the method of production, and they differ in the content of secondary plant metabolites, including polyphenols. This in turn affects the taste, texture, flavour, colour and stability of the wine. Most of the polyphenols are present in the grape skin and seeds. In red wine production, skins and stems are left in contact with the must for long periods of time, but for white wine production, stems, skins and must are separated soon after the juice extraction process.[15]

Recent studies performed on isolated rat hearts perfused with red wine extract before ischaemic arrest[22] have provided evidence that PACs from red wine are effective cardioprotective agents. The red wine extract reduced myocardial infarct size as well as improving post-ischaemic ventricular functions. In another study by the same group,[22] rats given oral PACs for three weeks were resistant to subsequent ischaemic injury to the isolated hearts.

Other research has shown that as well as acting as a cardioprotective agent directly, PACs also prevent atherosclerosis, which is a major risk factor for heart disease. It has been shown that *oxidation* of the polyunsaturated lipid components of LDL-C damages arteries and it is only this oxidised form of cholesterol that leads to atherosclerosis.[11] To determine whether the French paradox was due to the antioxidant properties of red wine, an *in vitro* study was carried out.[23] LDL-C from the blood of normolipidaemic, non-smoking volunteers was obtained by ultracentrifugation and diluted with buffered saline to a standard concentration of 1 mg/ml. Samples of the LDL-C were incubated for 2 hours with Californian red wine, from which all the ethanol had been removed by distillation, and copper sulfate, which catalyses the oxidation. Gas chromatography was then performed on the products formed. Comparison with authentic reference samples of pentane, hexanal and propanal, which are formed in the oxidation of polyunsaturated fatty acids, were used as a measure of the extent of oxidation. The polyphenolic samples caused an inhibition of 60% and 98% of the oxidation seen in the controls at concentrations of 3.8 mmol/L and 10 mmol/L respectively. When the phenolic samples were diluted 1000-fold with water, inhibition of oxidation was still seen. When the copper catalyst was used in excess, the antioxidant reaction was still effective, indicating that the reaction was not due to metal-chelating actions. These results show that the PACs in the red wine were acting as potent antioxidants, preventing the oxidisation of the LDL-C. It could well be that this is the explanation for the low levels of atherosclerosis seen in populations that consume large amounts of this drink.

A similar experiment was carried out recently using ten healthy volunteers.[24] First, samples of red and white wine were de-alcoholised and the fractions were tested for antioxidant activity. The red wine samples were 20 times more active than the white wine samples. Then at weekly intervals, the subjects drank 113 ml of the non-alcoholic component of red wine, white wine or tap water placebo. (Note that 113 ml of non-alcoholic wine were equivalent to 300 ml of alcoholic wine in terms of the phenolic compounds present.) Blood samples were taken before wine ingestion and at 30, 50 and 120 minutes after, and the total plasma antioxidant capacity was measured in a controlled peroxidation reaction. It was found that the antioxidant capacity of the plasma was significantly increased in those subjects who had ingested the non-alcoholic red wine, compared with non-alcoholic white wine or placebo. This indicated that the non-alcoholic fraction of red wine was indeed offering the antioxidant protection.

However, not all red wines have the same protective effect. It has been shown from research on more than 60 different red wines from 11 different countries that the PAC content and therefore the antioxidant properties vary greatly between different wines.[25] Red wines from Chile have a higher flavonol content than those from France, Italy, Australia and California. This could be due to differences in climate in the grape-growing regions, the thickness of the grape skins, the time of grape harvesting and the actual winemaking process, all of which could affect the flavonoid content.

It is worth noting that an alternative hypothesis has been suggested to account for the 'French paradox'. Several researchers claim that because until about 30 years ago France had a much healthier diet than now there has been a time lag in changes in the incidence of heart disease, similar to the time lag between smoking and lung cancer.[26] They propose that rather than being due to the red wine drunk in France, the difference in heart disease is due to these differences in diet. It is only in recent years that the French diet has become similar to that eaten in Britain and the USA, in terms of saturated fat and cholesterol intake. Only continued studies will show if this hypothesis is indeed correct. Even if this is the case, the research cited above strongly suggests that PACs, whether from red wine or other sources, certainly do offer protection against oxidation both *in vitro* and *in vivo*, and therefore play an important role in preventing heart disease.

It is interesting to note that many by-products of the wine industry are now being used in the nutraceutical industry; grape seeds and grape skins from winery waste in particular are being developed as dietary supplements.[27]

### *Direct inhibition of atherosclerosis by GSPE*

Although it has been presumed that the PACs protect against CVD by their antioxidant activity, most studies did not measure atherosclerosis directly. One *in vivo* study, however, did determine the effect of a PAC extract from grape seeds directly on atherosclerosis.[28] In this study, an extract containing 73.4% PAC was obtained by freeze-drying an aqueous solution of grape seeds. Thirty-eight rabbits were then fed with cholesterol and this extract or probucol (another type of antioxidant), for eight weeks, as shown in Table 4.4. Blood samples were withdrawn every two weeks and serum lipids and the lipoprotein components of the serum were measured enzymatically. The serum lipid profile did not change dramatically in the PAC-fed rabbits, but serum LDL-C and the LDL/HDL ratio decreased at six weeks in the 1% PAC group and HDL-C decreased at eight weeks in the 0.1% PAC group. Similarly, in the probucol group, total cholesterol and LDL-C values were lower than in the cholesterol-fed group.

The cholesterol contents of the aortic arch and the thoracic arch were also measured, as well as the percentage of the aortic surface area

**Table 4.4** The diets of the groups of rabbits used to determine the effect of cholesterol intake on atherosclerosis[28]

| *Group* | *Number* | *Standard diet* | *1% cholesterol* | *1% PAC* | *0.1% PAC* | *1% probucol* |
|---|---|---|---|---|---|---|
| 1 | 7 | + | | | | |
| 2 | 8 | + | + | | | |
| 3 | 8 | + | + | + | | |
| 4 | 8 | + | + | | + | |
| 5 | 7 | + | + | | | + |

PAC, proanthocyanidin.

covered with atherosclerotic lesions. There were similar levels of aortic plaque in both the probucol group and the PAC group, which were lower than in the cholesterol group (however, these were not reflected in the small changes in serum lipids measured). Probucol, 0.1% PAC and 1% PAC had all decreased the amounts of aortic plaque, but no dose-dependent activity was noted for the 0.1% and 1% PAC groups. PAC was not detected in serum or lipoproteins of the rabbits. The authors concluded that the PAC-rich extract inhibited the progression of atherosclerosis in cholesterol-fed rabbits. The activity of the PAC was thought to be related to prevention of LDL-C oxidation in the arterial cell wall.

## Vascular disorders

Another use for PACs that is widespread in Europe is in the treatment of vascular disorders. These include varicose veins, venous insufficiency and microvascular problems such as retinopathies. In France, PACs are the active ingredients in a proprietary product used for microcirculatory disorders called Endotelon. The antioxidant properties of the PACs are largely responsible for their vascular properties.[3]

### *A word of caution*

Although research has shown that antioxidants are beneficial to most people in preventing many different diseases, some trials have not produced the expected results. Some antioxidants act as pro-oxidants, depending on the timing of administration during oxidation processes and the individuals involved. It has been suggested that some individuals have higher rates of lipid peroxidation and are therefore at higher risk from diseases such as atherosclerosis and CVD, but in other individuals very high levels of antioxidants may actually cause pro-oxidation, worsening the damage. It may therefore be useful for populations to be screened to determine which people are at high risk and would benefit from antioxidants, rather than giving out a general recommendation for everyone to increase in their antioxidant intake.[29] This is an interesting viewpoint; however, the trials reviewed here indicate that in general antioxidants can be recommended, as such cases are rare.

## Prevention and treatment of cancer

At the start of the twenty-first century, the incidences of many degenerative diseases are increasing, even though huge advances in medical knowledge and technology have been made in the last decade. Cancer, for example, claims many lives, and vast resources of time, money and energy are being channelled into finding ways of reducing the risks. Although the best way to eliminate cancer is to prevent causative agents, such as cigarette smoking, in many cases the cause is unknown. In other cases neoplasia may have been initiated and the aim is to suppress the process. A large number of chemical compounds have been shown to prevent cancer by different mechanisms and at different stages in the neoplastic process[30] and the search for new agents continues.

It has been suggested that a diet rich in fruits and vegetables provides protection against tumour development. Geographical studies have shown that increased cancer risk is associated with high-fat/low-fibre diets, whereas diets based more on fruits and vegetables result in a much lower risk.[10] Phytochemicals such as PACs, which are widespread in fruits and vegetables, are an example of bioactive compounds that have been shown to reduce the risk of many types of cancer.

As discussed above, the PAC structure is based on the flavan-3-ol unit, which can be either *trans* (catechin) or *cis* (epicatechin). The monomers join together to form dimers, trimers and other oligomers, resulting in many different structures and functions, due to changes in stereochemistry. These structure–function relationships are very important in the quest for new anti-tumour agents. In one experiment, mice were used to assess the value of various PAC structures purified from Douglas fir bark. Three PAC dimers and an epicatechin trimer were investigated for anti-cancer activity and compared with the monomers, catechin and epicatechin, and with a control.[6] The isolated PACs were dissolved in acetone and applied to the shaved dorsal region of mice 15 minutes before the potent tumour promoter 12-O-tetradecanoylphorbol-13-acetate (TPA). Controls were prepared using acetone alone. The induction of ornithine decarboxylase (ODC) activity, stimulation of hydroperoxide production and increased DNA synthesis are biochemical events that are linked with TPA tumour promotion and were used to measure the inhibition of tumour promotion. (However, the respective responses to tumour promotion are not correlated and therefore orders of magnitude in the results varied, depending on which method was used.) In the induction of ODC activity, the epicatechin trimer showed the most inhibition (90%) compared with the dimers (56%) and monomers (35%). Hydroperoxide production was not inhibited by either monomer, but the dimers and trimer showed a 35–40% inhibition. In the inhibition of DNA synthesis all structures showed inhibition of 35–40%. The exact mechanism of tumour inhibition is unknown, but it could be connected to complex formation with the metal ions and cofactors required for the enzymic and non-enzymic generation of reactive oxygen species in multistage carcinogenesis. This might explain why the larger structures are more effective. In the case of DNA synthesis, all structures showed a similar degree of tumour inhibition, suggesting that other mechanisms are also involved.

In another study, fruit extracts of various *Vaccinium* species, which are high in PACs and other flavonoids, were screened for anti-tumour activity. Lowbush blueberry, bilberry, cranberry and lingonberry were fractionated by solvent partitioning and chromatographic methods and tested *in vitro*, using cultured mouse cells, for anti-cancer compounds.[31] Again, the greatest activity against TPA-induced carcinogenesis, measured by ODC inhibition, was found in the polymeric PAC fractions.

*In vitro* studies were also carried out to determine the effect of GSPE on human breast cancer cells, human lung cancer cells, human gastric adenocarcinoma cells and leukaemia cells.[32,33] The action of GSPE on normal human gastric mucosal cells was also assessed. When the cells were incubated with GSPE, concentration- and time-dependent inhibition was seen with the cancer cell lines, however the normal cells showed enhanced growth. Similarly, grape seed extracts have been shown to exhibit selective cytotoxicity against human oral tumour cell lines.[34]

These studies suggest that PACs in general and grape seed extract in particular, have a place in chemoprotection against cancer. More extensive work, including more *in vivo* testing and larger sample sizes, is required to provide conclusive evidence. It is certainly worth investigating whether these plant products have a place in the clinical prevention and treatment of cancer and so far the research seems promising.

It was previously thought that PAC extracts from various sources might be mutagens and induce liver tumours and oesophageal cancers.

The mutagenicity of several purified PACs, which included several dimers, a trimer and a polymer, was therefore tested on *Salmonella typhimurium* strains to see if these claims were founded.[35] None of the samples examined showed any mutagenic activity except PAC-B4, which is a dimer found in GSPE. Using high-performance liquid chromatography (HPLC) and thin-layer chromatography (TLC), it was discovered that the sample of B4 was contaminated with a mutagen called rutin that was identified using ultraviolet spectroscopy. Rutin is a flavonoid found in citrus fruit and has been reported to be of use in treating chronic venous oedema of the leg and leg oedema in pregnancy.[36,37] This study shows that rutin exhibits mutagenicity and it has been suggested that increased incidence of some tumours with flavonoids may be related to a balance of phase I enzymes which favour carcinogen activation rather than detoxification.[38] This result highlights the importance of using purified products and obtaining them from reliable sources. As the medical profession, as well as the public, become more aware of the availability and usefulness of nutraceuticals it is vital that the products offered by the industry are of the highest quality. As shown from this experiment, a contaminant can easily turn a phytochemical being promoted for its anti-tumour properties into a mutagen.

## Anti-viral agents

Viruses are responsible for many widespread diseases in both animals and plants. Just one example is the herpes simplex virus types 1 and 2, which cause stomatitis, meningitis and viral genital disease. Many research projects around the world are searching for pharmacological agents against such viruses and in particular against the human immunodeficiency virus (HIV). In a study to determine the structure–activity relationships of the anti-viral activity of various tannins,[39] it was found that the more condensed the structure the greater the anti-viral effect. It was therefore suggested that the active groups of polyphenols interact with the viral proteins and the host cell surface, causing decreased viral action and infection. The problem is that in many cases, anti-viral doses of polyphenols are similar to cytotoxic doses, making the use of PACs very limited.

In one study,[40] PACs were shown to have anti-herpes simplex virus activity. A cytotoxicity test was performed by adding thymidine to viral-infected cells *in vitro* and calculating the concentration necessary to decrease its uptake to 50% of the controls ($CC_{50}$). This was compared with the 50% effective dose ($EC_{50}$), needed to reduce herpes simplex plaque formation to 50% of controls. The $EC_{50}$ was found to be two to three orders of magnitude less than the $CC_{50}$. This shows that although there is some degree of toxicity, at the doses required for anti-viral action, the PACs were safe. Radioactively labelled viruses were used to show that the anti-herpes simplex effect was due to the inhibition of virus adsorption to the host cells.

The activity of *Piliostigma thonningii*, an African plant used in folk medicine to treat gum inflammation, against herpes simplex virus has been investigated. The purified root bark contains 10% epicatechin, 18% PAC-B2, 7% catechin trimers and other tetramers and oligomers based on the epicatechin structure. The purified polyphenolic fraction was used to test for anti-herpes simplex virus type 1 activity in African green monkey cells. The $EC_{50}$ was 17.5 μg/ml and the $CC_{50}$ was 44.8 μg/ml.[41] This result agrees with that reported above and shows that at doses required for anti-viral activity these PACs are only moderately cytotoxic.

Another *in vitro* experiment was carried out using the PAC from *Cupressus sempervirens* (CPAC) to determine anti-viral activity against the HIV and human T lymphotropic virus (HTLV) retroviruses.[42] These retroviruses are responsible for an attack on the immune system of the host organism, leading to increased susceptibility to infections, and they are sensitive to very few anti-viral agents. T lymphoblast and H9 cells were cultured and infected with HIV and HTLV respectively, at various concentrations. Each concentration was incubated with either the purified CPAC fraction or AZT (zidovudine), which is an anti-viral agent. The results showed that CPAC was more active against HIV than against HTLV. Concentrations of AZT necessary for the same amount of viral inhibition were much lower. However, AZT was found to be very cytotoxic even at very low concentrations, whereas CPAC showed negligible cytotoxicity at the $EC_{50}$ and could be used with no risk. Further studies *in vivo* are needed to determine whether this is a possible new use for PACs.

## Other uses

Plants have been used from ancient times to treat many different diseases. As the technology becomes available, many natural sources are being screened for isolated products with useful properties. The emphasis of these new agents must be on safety as well as efficacy, necessitating human studies. Many research teams are involved with purifying natural plant products in the search for novel uses and some of these are described below.

### *Chronic pancreatitis*

Two patients suffering from frequent abdominal pain arising from chronic pancreatitis were treated with 100 mg GSPE three times daily. In both cases the pain was greatly improved, even though previous medical therapy, including narcotic analgesics and pancreatic enzyme supplements, had failed to alleviate the symptoms.[43]

### *Hair growth*

Male baldness is a common condition for which treatments are continually being sought. In the 1980s, minoxidil, a drug prescribed for hypertension, was found to cause hair growth and thus became the first effective product licensed for this use. In an effort to discover other treatments, substances from the plant kingdom are often screened for activity in the hope of finding a cure for this widespread problem. One research team screened about 1000 different plant extracts from the roots, fruits, plants and seeds of 132 different plants in the search for a natural cure for male baldness.[44] The researchers found that the methanolic extract of grape seeds promoted hair follicle cell growth and PACs were identified as the active constituents. An *in vitro* study was then carried out using isolated and cultured mouse hair follicle cells. GSPE was found to increase hair growth in the cell culture by about 230%, compared with controls after five days and by 160% compared with minoxidil. An *in vivo* test was also performed using eight-week-old mice. The test substance was applied for 19 days to a shaven area on the backs of the mice. A 1% minoxidil solution resulted in 90–100% hair growth, 3% GSPE gave 80–90% growth and the control (vehicle only) resulted in 30–40% growth. No side-effects were seen in any group. From structure–function studies it was shown that the oligomers were more effective than monomers. The authors suggest that the PAC extract acts directly on the hair follicle cells, causing inhibition of cell differentiation and retention of the growing phase. These results indicate the possible use of GSPE in the treatment of baldness, but more extensive research is required, including human studies.

### *Natural sweeteners and the prevention of dental caries*

Sucrose, which is used extensively as a sweetener in foods, drinks and medicines because of its widespread availability and applications, is known to be the cause of dental caries. The enzyme glucosyltransferase, produced by bacteria on the teeth, is responsible for the development of dental caries from sucrose, via several intermediary stages.[45] Many foods are therefore sweetened with sugar alternatives. Other applications for alternative sweetening agents include diabetic foods and diet products, leading to a very large market for alternative sweeteners. Artificial sweeteners including saccharin and aspartame have been used for many years, but claims exist for possible toxicity and carcinogenicity.[46] Also, due to consumer demands for natural food ingredients, many plant compounds are already used as natural sweeteners in many countries, particularly in Japan, but concerns for their safety prevents licensing in other countries.

The search for new non-cariogenic, non-calorific sweeteners that can be used in diabetic preparations continues and to this end a team from Chicago isolated and purified many different plant compounds to test for possible new sweeteners.[46] A novel sweetener was isolated from the rhizomes of the fern *Selliguea feei*. The structure of this constituent was shown to be very similar to the typical PAC structure and showed lack of toxicity when fed to mice.

PACs are also known to prevent the development of dental caries by the inhibition of glucosyltransferase. The polyphenols in green and oolong tea have been shown to inhibit this enzyme and therefore prevent dental caries from forming. These mainly monomeric PACs have been used in foods and other products in Japan to prevent the occurrence of dental caries. PACs from bark extracts of several Japanese trees, which were mainly oligomeric, have also been reported to inhibit glucosyltransferase, with the inhibitory effect increasing as the size of the molecules increased.[45]

PACs are usually astringent when tasted and this finding necessitates more research into different PACs for their possible role as natural sweeteners. If a source of PACs that was both a natural sweetener and prevented dental caries could be isolated, this would be the ideal product.

### Cough suppressant

*Piliostigma thonningii* has been used in Africa for many years to treat coughs, lung diseases and gum inflammation. Until recently it was poorly investigated but research has shown a possible use as an anti-viral agent as described above. Isolated compounds, including epicatechin, PAC-B2, catechin trimers and oligomers, have been extracted from the plant. In one study,[47] anti-tussive activity was tested in guinea-pigs using codeine as a reference drug. In coughs induced by ammonia aerosol, both the extract and codeine reduced cough significantly. The extract was slightly less effective than codeine but the effect increased as the time between cough induction and extract delivery increased. With intravenous treatment the extract had a stronger effect than the codeine. Again, more research is required, but the folklore use does seem to be justified.

## Conclusions

The PACs, and more specifically grape seed proanthocyanidin extract, are showing some very interesting results in important health issues. More research is still required, particularly in the area of absorption and metabolism in human studies. The antioxidant properties of these supplements are well documented and *in vitro* and *in vivo* work in many areas shows that these non-essential nutrients could have a promising place in the treatment of diseases such as atherosclerosis, cancer and viral infections. However, large-scale human studies are lacking. Little information is available concerning side-effects or contraindications with other medications, although from toxicity studies[14] and from the other research reviewed here, PACs seem quite safe. As the understanding and use of antioxidants increases, it may well be found that this property is responsible for many other pharmacological uses of PACs in general and of GSPE in particular.

## References

1. Bagchi D, Garg A, Krohn R L *et al.* Protective effects of grape seed proanthocyanidins and selected antioxidants against TPA-induced hepatic and brain lipid peroxidation and DNA fragmentation, and peritoneal macrophage activation in mice. *Gen Pharmacol* 1998; 30: 771–776.
2. Haslam E. *Plant Polyphenols: Vegetable Tannins Revisited.* Cambridge: Cambridge University Press, 1989.
3. Fine A M. Oligomeric proanthocyanidin complexes: history, structure, and phytopharmaceutical applications. *Altern Med Rev* 2000; 5: 144–151.
4. Haslam E. Natural polyphenols (vegetable tannins) as drugs: possible modes of action. *J Nat Prod* 1996; 59: 205–215.
5. Da Silva Dias Duarte N M, do Nascimento J M. Pharmacological actions of proanthocyanidins. *Rev Port Farmac* 1998; 48: 9–12.
6. Gali H U, Perchellet E M, Gao X M, *et al.* Comparison of the inhibitory effects of monomeric, dimeric and trimeric procyanidins on the biochemical markers of skin tumour promotion in mouse epidermis *in vivo. Planta Med* 1994; 60: 235–239.
7. Evans W C. *Trease and Evans' Pharmacognosy*, 14th edn. London: W B Saunders, 1996.

8. Nigg H N, Seigler D. *Phytochemical Resources for Medicine and Agriculture*. New York: Plenum Press, 1992.
9. Mbwambo Z H, Luyengi L, Kinghorn A D. Phytochemicals; a glimpse into their structural and biological variation. *Int J Pharmacog* 1996; 34: 335–343.
10. German J B, Dillard C J. Phytochemicals and targets of chronic disease. In: Bidlack W R, Omaye S T, Meskin M S, Jahner D, eds. *Phytochemicals. A New Paradigm*. Pennsylvania: Technomic Publishing, 1998: 13–32.
11. Erasmus U. *Fats that Heal, Fats that Kill: the Complete Guide to Fats, Oils and Cholesterol*, 2nd edn. Burnaby BC, Canada: Alive Books, 1993.
12. Reiter R J. Cytoprotective properties of melatonin: presumed association with oxidative damage and ageing. *Nutrition* 1998; 14: 691–696.
13. Bagchi D, Garg A, Krohn R L, *et al.* Oxygen free radical scavenging abilities of vitamins C and E, and a grape seed proanthocyanidin extract *in vitro*. *Res Commun Mol Pathol Pharmacol* 1997; 95: 179–189.
14. Bagchi D, Bagchi M, Stohs S J, *et al.* Free radicals and grape seed proanthocyanidin extract: importance in human health and prevention. *Toxicology* 2000; 148: 187–197.
15. German J B, Walzem R L. The health benefits of wine. *Annu Rev Nutr* 2000; 20: 561–593.
16. Bagchi D, Kuszynski C, Balmoori J, *et al.* Hydrogen peroxide-induced modulation of intracellular oxidised states in cultured macrophage J7744A.1 and neuroactive PC-12 cells, and protection by a novel grape seed proanthocyanidin extract. *Phytother Res* 1998; 12: 568–571.
17. Davis W M. Antiaging products and tactics. *Drug Topics* 1997; 141; 92–101.
18. Bahorun T, Trotin F, Pommery J, *et al.* Antioxidant activities of *Crataegus monogyna* extracts. *Planta Med* 1994; 60: 323–328.
19. Renaud S, Lorgeril M. Wine, alcohol, platelets and the French paradox for coronary heart disease. *Lancet* 1992; 339: 1523–1526.
20. Rimm E B, Giovannucci E L, Willett W C, *et al.* Protective study of alcohol consumption and risk of coronary heart disease in men. *Lancet* 1991; 338: 464–486.
21. Lazarus N B, Kaplan G A, Cohen R D, *et al.* Change in alcohol consumption and risk of death from all causes and from ischaemic heart disease. *BMJ* 1991; 303: 553–556.
22. Das D K, Sato M, Ray P S, *et al.* Cardioprotection of red wine: role of polyphenolic antioxidants. *Drugs Exp Clin Res* 1999; 25: 115–120.
23. Frankel E N, Kanner J, German J B, *et al.* Inhibition of oxidation of human low-density lipoprotein by phenolic substances in red wine. *Lancet* 1993; 341: 454–457.
24. Serafini M, Maiani G, Ferro-Luzzi A. Alcohol-free red wine enhances plasma antioxidant capacity in humans. *J Nutr* 1998; 128: 1003–1007.
25. Anon. Not all red wines are equal, new research suggests. *Pharm J* 1999; 262: 213.
26. Law M, Wald N. Why heart disease mortality is low in France: the time lag explanation. *BMJ* 1999; 318: 1471–1480.
27. Shrikhande A J. Wine by-products with health benefits. *Food Res Int* 2000; 33: 469–474.
28. Yamakoshi J, Kataoka S, Koga T, *et al.* Proanthocyanidin-rich extract from

grape seeds attenuates the development of aortic atherosclerosis in cholesterol-fed rabbits. *Atherosclerosis* 1999; 142: 139–149.
29. Halliwell B. The antioxidant paradox. *Lancet* 2000; 355: 1179–1180.
30. Wattenberg L W. Chemoprevention of cancer. *Cancer Res* 1985; 45: 1–8.
31. Bomser J, Madhavi D L, Singletary K, *et al. In vitro* anticancer activity of fruit extracts from *Vaccinium* species. *Planta Med* 1996; 62: 212–216.
32. Joshi S S, Ye X, Liu W, *et al.* The cytotoxic effects of a novel grape seed proanthocyanidin extract on cultured human cancer cells. *Proc Am Assoc Cancer Res* 1998; 39: 227.
33. Ye X, Krohn R L, Liu W, *et al.* The cytotoxic effects of a novel IH636 grape seed proanthocyanidin extract on cultured human cancer cells. *Mol Cell Biochem* 1999; 196: 99–108.
34. Shirataki Y, Kawase M, Saito S, *et al.* Selective cytotoxic activity of grape peel and seed extracts against oral tumour cell lines. *Anticancer Res* 2000; 20: 423–426.
35. Yu C L, Swaminathan B. Mutagenicity of proanthocyanidins. *Food Chem Toxicol* 1987; 25: 135–139.
36. Clement D L. Management of venous oedema: insights from an international task force. *Angiology* 2000; 51: 13–27.
37. Young G L, Jewell D. Interventions for varicosities and leg oedema in pregnancy. *Cochrane Database Syst Rev* 2000; (2): CD001066.
38. Swanson C A. Vegetables, fruits, and cancer risk: the role of phytochemicals. In: Bidlack W R, Omaye S T, Meskin M S, Jahner D, eds. *Phytochemicals. A New Paradigm*. Pennsylvania: Technomic Publishing, 1998: 1–12.
39. Takechi M, Tanaka Y, Takehara M, *et al.* Structure and antiherpetic activity among the tannins. *Phytochemistry* 1985; 24: 2245–2250.
40. Fukuchi K, Sakagami H, Okuda T, *et al.* Inhibition of herpes simplex virus infection by tannins and related compounds. *Antiviral Res* 1989; 11: 285–298.
41. Cristoni A, Morazzoni P, Bombardelli E, *et al.* Activity of *Piliostigma thonningii* (Shum) root bark extract against herpes simplex virus type 1. *Phytother Res* 1996; 10: s135–s137.
42. Amouroux P, Jean D, Lamaison J L. Antiviral activity *in vitro* of *Cupressus sempervirens* on two human retroviruses HIV and HTLV. *Phytother Res* 1998; 12: 367–368.
43. Banerjee B, Trivedi M, Bagchi D. Beneficial effect of grape seed proanthocyanidin extract in the treatment of chronic pancreatitis. *Am J Gastroenterol* 1998; 93: 1653.
44. Takahashi T, Kamiya T, Yokoo Y. Proanthocyanidins from grape seeds promote proliferation of mouse hair follicle cells *in vitro* and convert hair cycle *in vivo*. *Acta Derm Venereol* 1998; 78: 428–432.
45. Mitsunaga T. Anti-caries activity of bark proanthocyanidins. *Basic Life Sci* 2000; 66: 555–573.
46. Kinghorn A D, Kaneda N, Baek N I, *et al.* Noncariogenic intense natural sweeteners. *Med Res Rev* 1998; 18: 347–360.
47. Bombardelli E, Lolla A, Pace R, *et al.* Proanthocyanidins from *Piliostigma thonningii*: chemical and pharmacological properties. *Planta Med* 1992; 58: A590.

# 5

# Lycopene

Lycopene is a natural red pigment synthesised by plants and micro-organisms, but not by animals. It is found in red fruits and vegetables, particularly the tomato, and is one of over 600 carotenoids found in nature; these function as pigments in photosynthesis and in photo-protection.[1–3] About 24 carotenoids are present in foods, including beta-carotene (found in carrots, broccoli and other green-leafed vegetables) and lutein (found in spinach, peas and watercress).[4] However, unlike many of the carotenoids, lycopene is not a precursor of vitamin A.

Research over the last ten years has shown possible useful activities of lycopene in several disease states, including the reduction of the risk of cancer and cardiovascular disease. Most studies used either dietary questionnaires to assess the intake of lycopene, or serum and adipose tissue concentrations, which were analysed by high-performance liquid chromatography (HPLC).

## Properties and structure

Most carotenoids have one- or two-ring structures, but lycopene ($C_{40}H_{56}$) is a linear structure and is an acyclic isomer of betacarotene (Figures 5.1 and 5.2). It is a highly unsaturated hydrocarbon with 11 conjugated and two unconjugated double bonds, normally all in the *trans* isomeric form, which is the most stable form. Chemical reactions, thermal energy and light all cause *cis–trans* isomerisation and in plasma it is present as an isomeric mixture. Lycopene is insoluble in water and is very hydrophobic.[1,2,5]

## Food sources and bioavailability

Tomatoes, watermelons, pink grapefruits and apricots as well as other red fruits and vegetables all contain lycopene (Table 5.1). Since humans are unable to synthesise carotenoids, there must be a sufficient intake from the diet. One group has estimated the usual dietary intake in Germany to be approximately 5 mg daily,[7] but others have estimated the

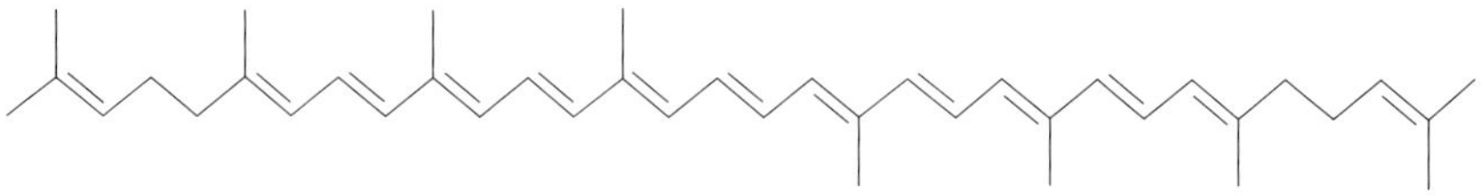

**Figure 5.1** The all-*trans* structure of lycopene.[1]

average daily intake in North America to be as high as 25 mg, with processed products accounting for at least 50% of the total intake. Based on these findings, the recommended daily intake has been set at about 35 mg, a value that is rarely met.[8]

Processed tomato products, such as tomato ketchup, tomato paste and tomato juice, are all good sources of lycopene and, unlike some other nutrients, lycopene is not lost through cooking or food processing. Indeed, the lycopene bioavailability increases with heat processing and therefore tomato-based products are often a better source than raw tomatoes (Table 5.1).[5]

Studies have shown that heat processing causes isomerisation of the ingested *trans*-lycopene to the *cis*- form, which may be responsible for the increased absorption.[8] Although most studies have been carried out using high-dose lycopene (16.5–75 mg/day), in a recent study using low-dose lycopene (5 mg/day) over a period of six weeks, it was found that both tomato juice and lycopene-containing soft gel capsules led to a higher absorption than fresh tomatoes.[7]

A lipid-rich diet also increases the bioavailability of lycopene and therefore the addition of oil to sauces and soups is beneficial. The presence of betacarotene and other carotenoids in the diet also enhance the bioavailability of lycopene and the carotenoids seem to act synergistically.[1,2] Once ingested, lycopene is found distributed non-uniformly in most human tissues; it concentrates in the adrenal glands, testes, liver and prostate.[2,5]

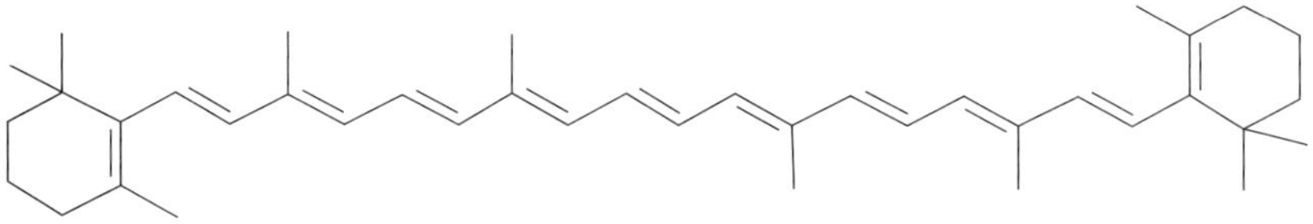

**Figure 5.2** Structure of betacarotene.[6]

**Table 5.1** Lycopene contents of some fruits and vegetables, including tomato-based products

| *Fruit/vegetable* | *Lycopene* ($\mu g/g$) |
|---|---|
| Watermelon | 23–72 |
| Pink guava | 54 |
| Pink grapefruit | 33.6 |
| Papaya | 20–53 |
| Apricot | <0.1 |
| Tomatoes (fresh) | 8.8–42 |
| Tomato products | |
| Tomato sauce | 62 |
| Tomato paste | 54–1500 |
| Tomato juice | 50–116 |
| Ketchup | 99–134.4 |
| Pizza sauce | 127.1 |

From ref. 5.

## Uses of lycopene

### Antioxidant

Most of the benefits of lycopene are probably due to its strong antioxidant action. (For a description of oxidation and antioxidation processes see Chapter 4.) Due to its strong hydrophobic nature, the reactions that occur only do so in a lipophilic environment.[5]

Early research into the properties of the carotenoids concentrated on betacarotene, which was found to be a good quencher of singlet oxygen ($^1O_2$), but lycopene was subsequently found to be an even stronger antioxidant.[9] The opening of the β-ionone ring to a linear chain seems to increase the antioxidant ability. The oxygen-quenching rate constant of lycopene *in vitro* was double that of betacarotene and 100 times that of α-tocopherol (vitamin E).[9] In other experiments, lycopene was again shown to be a better antioxidant than betacarotene and alphacarotene[6,10] and it also offered more protection to cells against photodynamic damage than betacarotene and other carotenoids.[11]

As well as singlet oxygen, lycopene has also been shown to quench other reactive species such as hydrogen peroxide, the species that generates the hydroxyl free radical (·OH), and also causes splitting of DNA strands[12] and nitrogen dioxide.[13] *In vivo* studies are required to determine whether these *in vitro* antioxidant reactions occur similarly in a clinical situation, but it seems likely that the antioxidant properties of lycopene confer its protective properties in many diseases, particularly in cancers, where oxidation reactions are known to be responsible for cellular damage.

## Cancer

Many epidemiologic studies have confirmed that a diet high in fruits and vegetables is associated with a decreased risk of various cancers. It has been suggested that 70% of all cancers can be attributed to diet,[5] and dietary antioxidants in particular are vital in protecting against many forms of this disease. Fruits and vegetables are high in many nutrients, including carotenoids, that act as powerful antioxidants and anti-tumour agents. Following advances in the technique of HPLC, the National Cancer Institute–US Department of Agriculture has been able to set up a database that specifies the carotenoid content of fruits and vegetables. Before this database was set up, it was wrongly assumed that betacarotene was the only carotenoid responsible for the cancer-preventative effects of diets rich in fruits and vegetables.[14]

### *Epidemiological studies*

Several papers have reviewed the epidemiological studies carried out on cancer and lycopene intake.[3,15] Lycopene was found to have a significant effect on the incidence of lung cancer in 10 out of 14 studies that assessed the association between tomato or lycopene intake and lung cancer. Most studies were adjusted for smoking, which is the highest risk factor for lung cancer and is the cause of more than 90% of all lung cancers. Stomach cancer, which remains one of the most common forms of cancer worldwide, was also inversely related to lycopene intake (12 studies). Low levels of lycopene have been observed in patients who developed cancers of the bladder (4 studies) and pancreas. Similarly, studies showed an inverse relationship between tomato-based products and the risk of colorectal cancer (5 studies), oral cancers (3 studies), oesophageal cancer (2 studies), pancreatic cancer (4 studies), prostate cancer (10 studies), breast cancer (4 studies, 3 or which showed a benefit) and cervical cancer (2 studies). Of the 72 studies that were included, 57 found inverse associations between tomato or lycopene intake or serum lycopene and risk of cancer, and 35 of these were statistically significant. Evidence was strongest for cancers of the lung, stomach and prostate and suggestive for cancers of the cervix, breast, colorectum, pancreas and oesophagus.

It must be remembered that tomatoes are also a very good source of vitamin C as well as folate, vitamin A and potassium, and they also contain other phytochemicals such as phenolic acids, phytosterols and flavonoids. Since purified lycopene extracts were not used in these studies, these other substances in addition to the lycopene may be contributing to the beneficial effects of the tomatoes and tomato-based products.[3,15]

Prostate cancer has been widely studied, as it is a very common form of cancer. As already mentioned, epidemiological evidence has shown that there is a marked reduction of prostate cancer risk in those consuming a diet high in lycopene. A study published in 1995[16] investigated the effect of different foods on the risk of prostate cancer. In 1986 the dietary intake of 47 894 subjects who were free of prostate cancer were assessed by a food-frequency questionnaire. Subsequently, additional questionnaires were sent to the same subjects in 1988, 1990 and 1992 and subjects were also asked whether there had been a diagnosis of prostate cancer in the previous two years. Altogether, 812 cases of prostate cancer were diagnosed by 1992. Of all the foods and food groups analysed from the questionnaires, four were significantly associated with lower risk and of these three were primary sources of lycopene, namely tomato sauce, tomatoes and pizza. (The fourth food was strawberries, in which the red colour is not due to lycopene.) Overall intake of vegetables was not associated with lowered risk and neither were carotenoids other than lycopene, including betacarotene, alphacarotene, lutein and β-cryptoxanthin.

In another study,[17] the serum and prostate-tissue lycopene concentrations were measured in 12 prostate cancer patients and compared with matched controls. Serum lycopene and prostate-tissue lycopene were both significantly lower in the cancer patients. These results again indicate the importance of lycopene in the risk of prostate cancer.

One study reported that increased tomato intake was related to a decrease in total cancer risk. The study was based on 42 cancer deaths in a population of 1271 elderly subjects. Other dietary factors associated with a low risk of cancer included green and yellow vegetables and strawberries.[18]

It is important to note that all studies were based on dietary intake and not on pharmacological doses of lycopene. Whether high or prolonged dosage would cause unwanted effects has not been determined and therefore only dietary lycopene can be recommended at this stage. Supplements may be required for those who do not like the taste of tomato products or who cannot eat them due to another adverse effect, such as allergy.

### *Animal studies*

The formation of colonic aberrant crypt foci (ACFs), which are precursors to colon cancer, were monitored in rats pre-treated with a carcinogen. The test groups also received alphacarotene, betacarotene, lycopene or lutein.[19] At low doses, alphacarotene, lycopene and lutein all inhibited the formation of ACFs, but betacarotene did not.

The effect of lycopene was studied in the induced rat mammary tumour.[20] The rats were treated with betacarotene or lycopene, starting two weeks before tumour induction at a dose of 10 mg/kg, twice weekly. The time from tumour induction until tumour appearance was measured in all groups (control – no injection, placebo – vehicle only injected, betacarotene and lycopene) and the rats were followed for four months. The number of tumours per rats' progress was highest at about 60% in the control group, as expected, but also in the betacarotene group. At the last time point the number and size of tumours was lowest in the lycopene group, even though both carotenoids had been well absorbed, and the difference was highly significant. It is interesting to note that, as in the previous study, betacarotene did not protect against tumour formation, whereas lycopene did so significantly.

The rat glioma-C6 cell line was derived from an induced rat brain tumour. These cells were then transplanted into male Wistar rats that were fed the same dose of various retinoids and carotenoids.[21] After approximately two months, the rats were killed and the tumours were removed and weighed. Both betacarotene and lycopene were potent inhibitors of tumour growth. Liver function tests showed that the retinoids and carotenoids used did not cause any abnormal liver functions.

### *Cell culture experimental studies*

At micromolar concentrations, lycopene inhibited the incorporation of [$^3$H] thymidine into Ishikawa endometrial cancer cells, lung cancer cells and mammary cancer cells in culture.[22] This showed that the lycopene had stopped the cancer cells from growing and this suppression of cell growth was secondary to inhibition of DNA synthesis. Lycopene was found to be a more potent inhibitor than either alphacarotene or betacarotene on the growth of these cancer cells. The researchers further showed that different lycopene preparations, including purified samples of lycopene, all inhibited cancer cell growth, which suggested that this was a direct action of lycopene rather than due to an unrelated contaminant.

In another experiment using cell cultures, lycopene caused a 40% reduction of growth of human promyelocytic leukaemia cell lines, compared with controls.[23]

## Cardiovascular disease

Cardiovascular disease (CVS) remains one of the most prevalent causes of mortality in both the developed world and in Third World countries. Known high-risk factors include smoking, diabetes, hypertension and hypercholesterolaemia. As described in Chapter 4, studies of lipid metabolism have shown that it is not the high cholesterol levels that cause atherosclerosis and CVS but rather the oxidised low-density lipoprotein cholesterol (LDL-C). The use of antioxidants would therefore be expected to reduce the incidence of CVS and this has been shown in epidemiological studies.[24]

The most widely studied carotenoid is betacarotene. A large, multicentre study ($n$ = 1410) showed that a high level of betacarotene from a normal diet, based on adipose tissue concentrations, was associated with a reduced risk of myocardial infarction, particularly in smokers.[25] However, further studies failed to show a reduction in CVS in smokers receiving betacarotene supplements and indeed suggested that supplements of betacarotene may be harmful in smokers, causing high mortality due to heart disease and lung cancer.[26] It was suggested that there might be other dietary contributions to the antioxidant effect seen from a diet high in fruits and vegetables, besides the effect of betacarotene.

Lycopene, often consumed with betacarotene, is one micronutrient that may be responsible for the protective effects noticed. In a large study carried out in ten different countries, the effects of alphacarotene, betacarotene and lycopene were studied in a population of men (average age 54 years) from coronary care units, who had undergone a first acute myocardial infarction.[24] The carotenoid concentration was measured from subcutaneous adipose tissue, since the adipose tissue levels of carotenoids are derived mainly from the diet and provide a better indication of dietary status than serum levels. Lycopene showed the greatest protective effect of the three carotenoids measured, after the results had been corrected for age, obesity, smoking and other risk factors.

Another study was carried out to determine why Lithuanian men have four times higher mortality from coronary heart disease than Swedish men do.[27] One hundred and one men aged 50 from Sweden, with no serious acute or chronic diseases, were compared with a similar population of 109 men from Lithuania. There were only small differences between the two groups in traditional risk factors (hypertension, smoking, high cholesterol levels), but when comparing the resistance of LDL to oxidation, a lower resistance was found in the men from Lithuania. There were also lower plasma concentrations of betacarotene, lycopene and $\gamma$-tocopherol in these men. These lower concentrations of antioxidants are due to the different diets of the two countries. It seems from this study that factors other than the usually cited risk factors are responsible for differences in mortality between Swedish and Lithuanian men. The antioxidant status may well account for these differences and, as already described, lycopene is one of the best dietary antioxidants and may therefore help to prevent CVS.

Oxidation of LDL-C is also associated with the formation of atherosclerotic plaques leading to strokes. Diets containing fruits and vegetables rich in antioxidants could therefore also offer protection against strokes. In a study of 26 593 male smokers aged 50–69 with no history of stroke in Finland, the subjects were asked to complete a detailed questionnaire about diet.[28] During a 6.1-year follow-up, 736 cerebral infarctions, 83 subarachnoid haemorrhages and 95 intracerebral haemorrhages occurred. The associations between these events and dietary intake were found to be significant only for betacarotene, but not for other nutrients, including flavonols, vitamin C, vitamin E, lutein and lycopene.

Although these reports suggest a beneficial effect of carotenoids and antioxidants on heart disease, and lycopene seems to be responsible for these outcomes, there is not yet conclusive evidence that lycopene itself contributes to the protective effects of fruit and vegetable consumption. A diet rich in fruits and vegetables, where many micronutrients are available to act synergistically, is therefore recommended at this stage, rather than individual supplements.

## Other uses

### *Age-related macular degeneration*

Age-related macular degeneration (ARMD) is the leading cause of irreversible blindness in elderly people. This disease affects 25% of people over 65 years old and is more common in women than in men. The macula is the central part of the retina and when it is damaged, the loss of central vision affects activities such as reading, driving and writing.[29,30] Although laser treatment has short-term benefits, there is no known cure for this disease at present. Dietary factors are now thought to help prevent or delay the onset of ARMD. A recent study compared the results of a food frequency questionnaire given to 356 subjects with advanced ARMD and 520 controls with other eye diseases, from five different ophthalmology centres.[30] It was found that those with a high carotenoid intake had a 43% lower risk of ARMD. This may be due to antioxidant effects, as the outer retina is rich in polyunsaturated fatty acids, which are very susceptible to oxidation, and is at high risk because of the exposure of the retina to light and oxygen. Another study[31] using 170 subjects assessed serum concentrations of several dietary antioxidants, including alphacarotene, betacarotene, lutein, lycopene, β-cryptoxanthin, α-tocopherol and γ-tocopherol. It was found that low levels of lycopene were related to an increased possibility of having ARMD. Further clinical studies would be useful to provide more evidence in this field.

### *Functional status*

As ageing progresses, there is often an accompanying decreased ability to perform normal daily functions, such as bathing, dressing, walking, eating and drinking. This may be caused by the accumulation of oxidative damage, leading to a decline in functional status.[32] In an epidemiological study carried out on a population of 88 elderly Roman Catholic nuns, blood samples were taken and the subjects were assessed for mental and physical function.[32] The blood was analysed for various antioxidants, including carotenoids, as well as for blood lipids and albumin. Results showed a strong correlation between lycopene and the ability to self-care, which was not evident with other antioxidants. This preliminary study suggests that there may be a link between serum lycopene and functional status. Repetition of the study in other populations is necessary before any definite conclusions can be reached. Low serum lycopene may just reflect excessive oxidation and therefore studies assessing the lycopene intake rather than plasma concentration with function would be beneficial.

## Mechanisms of action

Unlike other carotenoids, such as betacarotene, whose cancer-protective properties are based on a combination of antioxidant effects and conversion to vitamin A, lycopene is not a precursor of vitamin A and therefore other mechanisms of action have been sought, in addition to the widely accepted action of antioxidant. These will be considered below.

## Antioxidant

It has been suggested that the carotenoids confer their anti-cancer effects by deactivating certain reactive molecular species, preventing cellular damage and breaking the damaging chain reaction that ultimately leads to cancer.[18] Unlike betacarotene, because it is not converted to vitamin A, lycopene is entirely available as an antioxidant. The conjugated structure enables the molecule to absorb light and to inactivate singlet oxygen and free radicals. Also the lack of the β-ionone ring increases its antioxidant activity. Stereochemically, lycopene differs from other carotenoids, making it uniquely present in some cellular environments. It is therefore able to act as an antioxidant, protecting the cells against damage from smoking, sunlight, chronic inflammation and normal metabolic processes.[15] Oxidation can cause damage to the unsaturated phospholipid membrane, which causes tumour-promoting products, and oxidative damage to DNA can produce mutagens.[33]

## Suppression of IGF-1

As well as antioxidant properties, lycopene also affects the insulin-like growth factor 1 (IGF-1)-stimulated growth of cancer cells. Cancer cells grow so quickly partly due to the augmented secretion of growth factors. Lycopene inhibited the growth due to IGF-1 in an experiment using endometrial cancer cells.[22] The IGF system is very complex, including two different growth factors and many receptors and the precise action of lycopene on the suppression of this mechanism of cancer growth has yet to be confirmed.

## Gap junction communication

The mouse embryo fibroblast C3H/10T1/2 cell line was used to show that lycopene acts by upregulating gap communication between cells. Gap junctional communication is an important part of cell growth control and carcinogenesis. Tumour promoters inhibit this communication and disrupt normal cell growth, whereas agents that enhance cell–cell communication lead to increased growth of normal cells and malignant cells, but suppression of transformation of carcinogen-initiated cells, which is an important stage in carcinogenesis.[33]

### Metabolic pathways

In an animal experiment using rat liver carcinogenesis, one of the best models to test the effect of carcinogens on the different stages of carcinogenesis,[34] lycopene significantly decreased the size of liver preneoplastic foci (which are precursors to liver cancer) and of the fraction of the liver occupied by such foci induced by the carcinogen diethylnitrosamine (DEN) in the initiation phase of liver cancer. The mechanisms of action appeared to be related to the metabolic pathways rather than antioxidant effects. DEN acts through the cytochrome P-450 pathway and it would seem that lycopene interfered with cancer initiation via this pathway.

One research team found that lycopene contributed to a minor hypocholesterolaemic effect in six healthy volunteers over three months.[35] The mechanism for this action was related to the synthetic pathway that lycopene shares with cholesterol and the ability of lycopene to inhibit macrophage 3-hydroxy-3-methyl glutarate coenzyme A (HMG-CoA), which is the rate-limiting enzyme in cholesterol biosynthesis.

### Immune function

Stimulation of T lymphocytes by antigen-presenting cells leads to cell-mediated immune responses. This mechanism is involved in the immune response to infections and neoplastic cells. Some carotenoids enhance this cell-mediated response by enhancing the expression of the cell surface molecules, as demonstrated by a study in which healthy non smokers given betacarotene (15 mg/day) for 26 days, showed enhanced cell-mediated responses.[4] In a similar study using 23 subjects given either a lycopene-rich tomato extract or a lutein-rich marigold extract for 26 days, although some immune-function enhancement was seen, there was a less marked effect in either case compared with the earlier study with betacarotene. This may have been related to the lower plasma levels of these two carotenoids after supplementation compared with those measured after betacarotene supplementation.[4] This study showed that different carotenoids have different effects on the immune system and it cannot be assumed that the effect of one carotenoid will be the same as another. Further studies are required to see if different intakes or synergistic effects with other plant nutrients would increase the immune enhancement of lycopene.

In one study in which elderly subjects were given fruit and vegetable extract supplements containing multiple antioxidants and phytonutrients for 80 days, there was a significant improvement in immune function. The extracts included apple, orange, pineapple, papaya, cranberry, peach, carrot, parsley, beet, broccoli, kale, cabbage, spinach and tomatoes.[36]

A combination of mechanisms including inhibition of oxidative damage to DNA and membrane phospholipids, induction of cell–cell communication, growth control and enhanced cell-mediated immunity are therefore responsible for the anti-cancer properties of this important carotenoid.[3]

## Conclusions

Although there are many epidemiological studies and much evidence to suggest that lycopene is beneficial in preventing cancers and other diseases, there are very few human clinical trials. Animal experiments and cell culture studies show promising results but the value of lycopene in disease remains suggestive rather than conclusive.

The general recommendation to increase the intake of fruits and vegetables in general and tomato-based products in particular is therefore favoured over supplementation with lycopene alone. The resulting dietary increase of mixed carotenoids as well as many other phytonutrients leads to a synergistic effect and is preferable at this stage until more definite conclusions can be reached about the specific value of lycopene.

## References

1. Agarwal S, Rao A V. Tomato lycopene and its role in human health and chronic diseases. *Can Med Assoc J* 2000; 163: 739–744.
2. Bramley P M. Is lycopene beneficial to human health? *Phytochemistry* 2000; 54: 233–236.
3. Sengupta A, Das S. The anti-carcinogenic role of lycopene, abundantly present in tomato. *Eur J Cancer Prev* 1999; 8: 325–330.
4. Hughes D A, Wright A J A, Finglas P M, *et al.* Effects of lycopene and lutein supplementation on the expression of functionally associated surface molecules on blood monocytes from healthy male non-smokers. *J Infect Dis* 2000; 182(suppl 1): S11–S15.
5. Rao A V, Agarwal S. Role of lycopene as antioxidant carotenoid in the prevention of chronic diseases: a review. *Nutr Res* 1999; 19: 305–323.
6. Miller N J, Sampson J, Candeias L P, *et al.* Antioxidant activities of carotenes and xanthophylls. *FEBS Lett* 1996; 384: 240–242.
7. Bohm V, Bitsch R. Intestinal absorption of lycopene from different matrices and interactions to other carotenoids, the lipid status, and the antioxidant capacity of human plasma. *Eur J Nutr* 1999; 38; 118–125.

8. Rao A V, Agarwal S. Role of antioxidant lycopene in cancer and heart disease. *J Am Coll Nutr* 2000; 19: 563–569.
9. Mascio P, Kaiser S, Sies H. Lycopene as the most efficient biological carotenoid singlet oxygen quencher. *Arch Biochem Biophys* 1989; 274: 532–538.
10. Mortensen A, Skibsted L H. Relative stability of carotenoid radical cations and homologue tocopherol radicals. A real time kinetic study of antioxidant hierarchy. *FEBS Lett* 1997; 417: 261–266.
11. Tinkler J H, Bohm F, Schalch W, *et al.* Dietary carotenoids protect human cells from damage. *J Photochem Photobiol B: Biol* 1994; 26: 283–285.
12. Lu Y, Etoh H, Watanabe N, *et al.* A new carotenoid, hydrogen peroxide oxidation products from lycopene. *Biosci Biotechnol Biochem* 1995; 59: 2153–2155.
13. Mortensen A, Skibsted L H, Sampson J, *et al.* Comparative mechanisms and rates of free radical scavenging by carotenoid antioxidants. *FEBS Lett* 1997; 418: 91–97.
14. Heber D. Colourful cancer prevention: α-carotene, lycopene, and lung cancer. *Am J Clin Nutr* 2000; 72: 901–902.
15. Giovannucci E. Tomatoes, tomato-based products, lycopene, and cancer: review of the epidemiologic literature. *J Natl Cancer Inst* 1999; 91: 317–331.
16. Giovannucci E, Ascherio A, Rimm E B, *et al.* Intake of carotenoids and retinol in relation to risk of prostate cancer. *J Natl Cancer Inst* 1995; 87: 1767–1776.
17. Rao A V, Fleshner N, Agarwal S. Serum and tissue lycopene and biomarkers of oxidation in prostate cancer patients: a case-control study. *Nutr Cancer* 1999; 33: 159–164.
18. Colditz G A, Branch L G, Lipnick R J, *et al.* Increased green and yellow vegetable intake and lowered cancer deaths in an elderly population. *Am J Clin Nutr* 1985; 41: 32–36.
19. Narisawa T, Fukaura Y, Hasebe M, *et al.* Inhibitory effects of natural carotenoids, α-carotene, β-carotene, lycopene and lutein, on colonic aberrant crypt foci formation in rats. *Cancer Lett* 1996; 107: 137–142.
20. Sharoni Y, Giron E, Rise M, *et al.* Effects of lycopene enriched tomato oleoresin on 7,12-dimethyl-benz[a]anthracene-induced rat mammary tumours. *Cancer Detect Prev* 1997; 21: 118–123.
21. Wang C J, Chou M Y, Lin J K. Inhibition of growth and development of the transplantable C-6 glioma cells inoculated in rats by retinoids and carotenoids. *Cancer Lett* 1989; 48: 135–142.
22. Levy J, Bosin E, Feldman B, *et al.* Lycopene is a more potent inhibitor of human cancer cell proliferation than either α-carotene or β-carotene. *Nutr Cancer* 1995; 24: 257–266.
23. Countryman C, Bankson D, Collins S, *et al.* Lycopene inhibits the growth of the HL-60 promyeloctic leukemia cell line. *Clin Chem* 1991; 37: 1056.
24. Kohlmeier L, Kark J D, Gomez-Gracia E, *et al.* Lycopene and myocardial infarction risk in the EURAMIC study. *Am J Epidemiol* 1997; 146: 618–626.
25. Kardinaal A F M, Kok F J, Ringstad J, *et al.* Antioxidants in adipose tissue and risk of myocardial infarction: the EURAMIC study. *Lancet* 1993; 342: 1379–1384.
26. The Alpha-tocopherol, Beta Carotene Cancer Prevention Study Group. The

effect of vitamin E and beta carotene on the incidence of lung cancer and other cancers in male smokers. *N Engl J Med* 1994; 330: 1029–1035.

27. Kristenson M, Zieden B, Kucinskiene A, *et al.* Antioxidant state and mortality from coronary heart disease in Lithuanian and Swedish men: concomitant cross sectional study of men aged 50. *BMJ* 1997; 314: 629–633.
28. Hirvonen T, Virtamo J, Korhonen P, *et al.* Intake of flavonoids, carotenoids, vitamins C and E, and risk of stroke in male smokers. *Stroke* 2000; 31: 2301–2306.
29. Regtop H. Age related macular degeneration. *Aust J Med Herbalism* 1998; 10: 38–45.
30. Seddon J M, Ajani U, Sperduto R D, *et al.* Dietary carotenoids, vitamins A, C and E, and advanced age-related macular degeneration. *JAMA* 1994; 272: 1413–1420.
31. Mares-Perlman J A, Brady W E, Klein R, *et al.* Serum antioxidants and age-related macular degeneration in a population-based case-control study. *Arch Ophthalmol* 1995; 113: 1518–1523.
32. Snowdon D A, Gross M D, Butler S M. Antioxidants and reduced functional capacity in the elderly: findings from the nun study. *J Gerontol* 1996; 51A: M10–M16.
33. Zhang L X, Cooney R V, Bertram J S. Carotenoids enhance gap junctional communication and inhibit lipid peroxidation in C3H/10T1/2 cells: relationship to their cancer chemopreventive action. *Carcinogenesis* 1991; 12: 2109–2114.
34. Astorg P, Gragelet S, Berges R, *et al.* Dietary lycopene decreases the initiation of liver preneoplastic foci by diethylnitrosamine in the rat. *Nutr Cancer* 1997; 29: 60–68.
35. Fuhrman B, Elis A, Aviram M. Hypocholesterolemic effect of lycopene and β-carotene is related to suppression of cholesterol synthesis and augmentation of LDL receptor activity in macrophages. *Biochem Biophys Res Commun* 1997; 233: 658–662.
36. Inserra P F, Jiang S, Solkoff D, *et al.* Immune function in elderly smokers and nonsmokers improves during supplementation with fruit and vegetable extracts. *Integrative Med* 1999; 2: 3–10.

# 6

# Carnitine

Carnitine (3-hydroxy-4-*N*-trimethylaminobutyric acid) is an essential cellular component, synthesised from the essential amino acids lysine and methionine in the liver and kidney, from where it is released into the systemic circulation. It is also synthesised in the brain.[1–3] Although it was originally shown to be an essential nutrient for the worm *Tenebrio molitor* and was referred to as vitamin $B_T$, it is now not considered to be a vitamin but rather a 'vitamin-like substance'.[4] Carnitine is widely used in carnitine-deficiency conditions, and in many countries in Europe (including Britain) L-carnitine is frequently prescribed.[5] The other main use is as a dietary supplement for various diseases and in some countries it is available without a prescription for this purpose.

## Properties and structure

Carnitine exists in two isomeric forms, the D- and L-forms. The two forms have different biochemical and pharmacological properties. Naturally occurring carnitine is almost always the L-isomer, whereas the D-isomer is usually synthetic. The L-isomer is a substrate for carnitine acetyltransferase and is the only isomer with biological activity, but the D-isomer acts as a competitive inhibitor, interfering with fatty acid oxidation and energy production.[4] Some patients find it difficult to excrete the D-isomer and it has also been reported that administration of the D-isomer led to a depletion of L-carnitine in the heart muscle, leading to abnormalities.[2] D-Carnitine and DL-carnitine are therefore toxic and not safe for human consumption and have been banned in the USA.[4] For the purposes of this review the L-isomer only has been considered (Figure 6.1).

Cofactors required for the biosynthesis of carnitine include vitamin C, niacin, pyridoxal 5-phosphate (vitamin $B_6$), magnesium and iron. Ninety-eight per cent of carnitine is found in the cardiac and skeletal muscle, with a further 1.5% in liver and kidneys and 0.5% in extracellular fluid. Carnitine can also be obtained from the diet, predominantly from food of animal origin, such as meat and dairy produce. In humans,

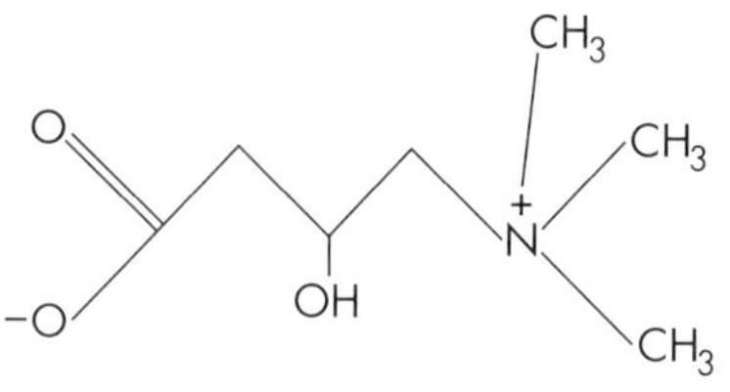

**Figure 6.1** Structure of carnitine.[3]

100–200 μmol carnitine is synthesised daily and a normal diet contains approximately 300–400 μmol daily.[6] Some researchers have reported an oral bioavailability of between 54% and 87%,[7] but others suggest much lower bioavailability, of about 18%.[8] Although the amount ingested determines the absorption rate, oral doses of greater than 2 g have no advantage, since at this dose mucosal absorption seems to be saturated.[3] In vegetarians, metabolic needs are usually met by endogenous biosynthesis.[9] Carnitine levels would have to drop by more than 50% to lead to a marked metabolic change, and this does not usually occur even in strict vegetarians.[4] Plasma carnitine levels are higher in males than in females, and older females (above 40 years) have lower levels still.[1,2]

## Metabolism

The main function of carnitine is in fatty acid (FA) metabolism. The biochemical reactions of this nutrient are based on the reversible reaction between carnitine and long-chain FA acyl groups:

$$\text{Carnitine} + \text{Acyl CoA} \Leftrightarrow \text{Acyl carnitine} + \text{Coenzyme A}$$

Carnitine is therefore involved with many coenzyme A-dependent pathways.[10] The first recognised function of carnitine was the involvement in long-chain FA oxidation, at the mitochondrial level, providing energy. Carnitine acts as a carrier of the acyl and acetyl groups across the mitochondrial membrane. Once inside the mitochondria, β-oxidation can occur to provide energy from the long-chain FAs.[11] This is the main energy source in skeletal and cardiac muscle, attesting to the important role of carnitine.[3] When acetyl formation exceeds the amount needed in the Krebs cycle, it is transported out of the mitochondria as acetyl CoA. It is now known that carnitine is also involved in many other metabolic functions. These include the metabolism of branched chain α-keto acid oxidation and detoxification of potentially toxic acyl CoA metabolites from other pathways.

A small amount of carnitine is excreted by the kidneys in the urine as free carnitine or as acyl carnitine, but more than 85% is reabsorbed by the proximal renal tubule.[1,12]

## Deficiency syndromes

When carnitine levels are very low, there is an accumulation of free FAs in the cell cytoplasm and an excess of acyl CoA in the mitochondria. This leads to altered energy production from FAs.[1] Deficiency in those on a normal diet is rare, although there has been a report of carnitine deficiency resulting from a strict vegetarian diet.[13] A deficiency of any of the cofactors that are necessary for the biosynthesis of carnitine, such as iron, vitamin C and vitamin $B_6$ may also have an effect on carnitine levels.[3] Moreover, deficiency can occur due to a primary cause, such as an inborn error of metabolism, or secondary either to another disease or to drug administration (described below). Inadequate intake or excessive loss can result in very low carnitine levels, but this does not necessarily lead to clinical symptoms.[9] In the new-born, FA oxidation is very important to provide the energy required for rapid growth, and in preterm infants carnitine biosynthesis may be inadequate for the needs of the baby due to immature enzyme systems. In these cases, carnitine supplementation may be of benefit to improve growth, especially in those babies who have to be fed with intravenous solutions that do not contain carnitine.[14]

Clinical symptoms of carnitine deficiency, whether primary or secondary, can manifest in two ways. In adults, carnitine deficiency usually presents as chronic muscle weakness due to muscle carnitine deficiency.[2] In infants and young children, carnitine deficiency leads to repeated bouts of coma, hypotonia, muscle weakness, recurrent infections, hypoglycaemia and a Reye's-like syndrome (Reye's syndrome involves acute encephalopathy and the fatty degeneration of the liver, and has been associated with giving aspirin to children). Treatment is required to restore carnitine levels to 20 μmol/L, using doses of 100–600 mg/kg daily. There have been several reports of carnitine supplementation in such cases, but due to the problems of setting up clinical trials for children with metabolic disorders, most accounts have been single-case reports or anecdotal. In some reports patients with lethal metabolic disorders have exceeded their predicted lifespan and developed remarkably in response to carnitine.[15,16] In a study carried out on malnourished Turkish children aged 9–18 months suffering from kwashiorkor (limited protein intake) and marasmus (limited calorie intake) it was found that these children had significantly lower carnitine levels compared with healthy children from the same community. Sixteen out of the 41 malnourished children were randomly chosen for carnitine supplementation at a dose of 100 mg/kg/day. After only five days of supplementation, carnitine levels returned to normal and continued carnitine administration did not increase the levels further. This may be a novel way to increase growth in children with malnutrition.[17]

## Uses of carnitine

### Athletic performance

As already described, carnitine is involved with fatty acid oxidation, which provides energy, and also in the transport of acyl groups from the mitochondria. Since both of these actions are required for peak exercise performance and training, it is logical to hypothesise that carnitine may be of value as a supplement for sportsmen/women, who are constantly looking for new (and legal) ways to enhance their performance. Since endogenous carnitine pools are large (approximately 20 g in a 70-kg healthy man) and bioavailability studies have reported the oral bioavailability to vary from approximately 15% to 85%, it is difficult to determine how much carnitine is being absorbed from any particular dose. A long duration of study is also important to reach maintained increases in the carnitine pool. Reviews of recent clinical trials[4,9,18] showed that although some studies were favourable, many others were not. There were drawbacks in the experimental design of many of the trials, including variations of route, dose and duration of treatment, with a length of only one or two weeks in most trials. Moreover, most of the trials cited used small numbers of subjects. The endpoints used also varied between performance-based endpoints and metabolic measurements. In exercise performance experiments, it is also important to have a sufficiently long wash-out period in crossover trials, and in some of the published trials this was not the case. Several long-term studies have also been reported, again with equivocal results.[4]

There have been some promising reports of the use of carnitine in aerobic sports,[19] and for preventing muscle damage during strenuous exercise, especially in untrained athletes. One study also showed that carnitine improved recovery time in nine out of twelve healthy, young subjects after strenuous exercise.[4] Moreover, carnitine supplementation may be beneficial in exercise performance in disease states, such as chronic renal failure and peripheral vascular disease.[18] It has been suggested that carnitine supplementation only results in a significant advantage for sportsmen/women in cases where there was a deficiency beforehand.[3] At present, however, carnitine cannot be recommended as an ergogenic agent for healthy athletes and sportsmen/women. Further clinical trials involving large groups of subjects and long periods of carnitine therapy are required to determine whether carnitine will have a role as an ergogenic agent in the future.

## Haemodialysis patients

End-stage renal disease is fatal unless there is either a kidney transplant or long-term haemodialysis (HD). Side-effects of HD include anaemia, compromised heart function and depression, which in turn leads to poor compliance and worsening of symptoms. Carnitine supplementation has recently been investigated in HD and found to improve many of these problems in long-term HD patients.

Since the 1970s, it has been known that carnitine levels are altered in chronic renal failure and in HD patients. Reasons for this include decreased intestinal uptake, especially in patients with a low protein diet, and decreased biosynthesis, as well as the loss of carnitine through HD.[6] One of the cofactors necessary for carnitine biosynthesis, palmitoyl transferase, is reduced in chronic renal failure, which may be a cause of a decline in biosynthesis. There have been many studies investigating the effect of carnitine on anaemia in HD, which have been reviewed in the literature.[1,4] Early studies did not always differentiate between total and free plasma carnitine, leading to conflicting results. In recently published studies, total carnitine levels of plasma before dialysis were equal to or higher than controls, but free carnitine levels were decreased. This indicates that renal failure affects the free carnitine levels, rather than total carnitine levels, and care must be taken when interpreting results and comparing different studies.[1]

### *Erythropoietin dose*

As stated above, in chronic renal failure patients on HD, anaemia is frequently a problem. This is usually due to decreased red blood cell (RBC) production by the diseased kidney. Recombinant human erythropoietin (rHuEPO) is often used to treat these patients, but is very costly. Several factors can affect the dose of rHuEPO required, including blood loss, iron deficiency, aluminium toxicity, inflammation, infection and malignancy.[20,21] However, because the treatment is so expensive, rHuEPO is not usually started until the haematocrit (the proportion of circulating blood occupied by RBCs) falls below about 30%, which is much lower than the normal level of 37–50%. Many patients receiving rHuEPO have low carnitine levels, and this has also been shown to affect the amount of rHuEPO needed.[20] Fourteen HD patients who showed a poor response to rHuEPO were included in one recent study.[21] Haematocrit levels were less than 27.5% despite a weekly dose of 9000 U rHuEPO for three months, and none of the factors (listed above) that affect the dose required were present. All of the subjects received 500 mg carnitine orally each day for three months. Results showed significant increases in haematocrit. The study also found that serum carnitine levels varied significantly between those patients who maintained haematocrit levels of above 30% without rHuEPO, and those requiring it. This strongly suggests that carnitine supplementation is beneficial in those undergoing HD, especially where rHuEPO is indicated but there is a poor response, or indeed to lower the dose of rHuEPO required.

In a similar placebo-controlled, randomised, double-blind study,[1] 40 HD patients were given either carnitine or placebo after each dialysis session, for eight months. For the first four months, 20 mg intravenous iron was also administered after each session, as iron deficiency has also been implicated in failure of rHuEPO. As in the previous experiment, rHuEPO dose was adjusted according to haematocrit values. Results showed that at the end of the study period, most of the subjects still had free carnitine levels below the reference range for healthy subjects. The rHuEPO dose was reduced as a result of carnitine administration in the first four months, but when iron therapy was discontinued the rHuEPO requirement increased in both groups, suggesting that iron as well as carnitine is necessary to improve the anaemia of HD.

Interestingly, a small ($n$ = 16) study in children failed to show a similar significant change in rHuEPO requirement when carnitine supplementation was given for 26 weeks,[22] which contrasts with the adult studies.

### *Elderly dialysis patients*

As well as chronic renal failure, ageing also leads to a reduction of carnitine and of erythropoietin, which are both synthesised by the kidney.

Therefore a randomised, double-blind study was carried out to determine the benefit of carnitine in older dialysis patients.[23] Thirty-one patients aged between 41 and 95 were selected. They had all been receiving HD for more than one year and rHuEPO for at least nine months, and had haematocrit values between 30% and 35%, but iron levels were normal. The subjects received either 1 g intravenous carnitine at the end of each dialysis session, or placebo, for six months. The rHuEPO dose was adjusted every two weeks, corresponding to the individual blood profile. Plasma carnitine levels were measured before the study, and after three and six months of starting the treatment. The results showed a reduced need for rHuEPO in the patients receiving carnitine supplementation, and/or improved haematocrit values without the need for increasing the rHuEPO dose, with the best results in those patients over 65 years of age. Decreasing rHuEPO dosage with the use of carnitine therapy could lead to considerable financial savings, which would enable rHuEPO to be given before clinical symptoms of anaemia are reached. This could have far-reaching consequences, particularly in the elderly population that is sometimes denied expensive treatments.

### *Dialysis patients with heart disease*

Carnitine deficiency in long-term dialysis patients can also lead to cardiac problems, which can be severe. Since carnitine is required for the transport of FAs for energy production, if carnitine levels are reduced, the heart muscle cannot produce energy and cardiac function is compromised. Hence cardiac disease is the main cause of mortality in HD patients.[24] A small clinical study was carried out using 11 patients who had been receiving HD for between 11 and 30 years, compared with eight controls with neither renal nor cardiac disease.[25] Carnitine was taken orally (1 g/day for the first month and 0.5 g/day for a second month). Before the study was started, both total and free carnitine levels in the dialysis patients were lower than in the controls, as expected. After the two months of carnitine supplementation, both total and free carnitine plasma levels increased significantly in the patients, exceeding those of the controls. The defective myocardial fatty acid metabolism observed before the treatment period, which can eventually lead to heart failure in chronic renal patients, was also corrected, suggesting another advantage for carnitine supplementation in HD patients.

In another small clinical study nine HD patients were selected, who also showed signs of left ventricular hypertrophy and who had suffered from chest symptoms for at least three months.[24] Patients received 500 mg carnitine daily for six months. Chest pain and palpitations were markedly ameliorated by the carnitine treatment, and cardiac function was also improved.

### *Quality of life*

As well as cardiac problems, long-term HD often leads to a reduced quality of life resulting from weakness, tiredness and a general decrease in energy metabolism. Since carnitine is involved in energy metabolism, a trial was carried out to determine whether carnitine supplementation would alter patients' perceived quality of life.[26] One hundred and one patients were included in the study and divided into three groups. Group one received 1 g carnitine orally, before and after each dialysis treatment, for six months; group two received placebo; and group three received three months of placebo followed by three months of carnitine, or vice versa. Every six weeks, the patients had to fill out a questionnaire assessing various parameters associated with quality of life. These were bodily pain, emotional role, general health, mental health, physical function (limits to physical activities), physical role (physical limits to daily activities), social function and vitality. Since diabetes and hypertension are often causes of renal disease, results were compared with these populations. A questionnaire was also completed at the end of each dialysis session, reporting any symptoms associated with the dialysis itself, such as chest pain, headache, nausea and muscle cramps. These values were not affected by the carnitine therapy. Except for physical role, quality of life assessments were perceived as low in the HD patients, compared with healthy subjects or those with diabetes or hypertension, before the study was started. After three months, carnitine patients reported an increase in vitality and general health and after six months physical function also improved, but some patients' perception of mental health and vitality was again lower. In other words, the initial benefits in quality of life were not maintained for more than 1.5–3 months of treatment. This could be due to the plateau reached which is perceived as a decrease in some subjects, because they expected an improvement. Alternatively, long-term carnitine therapy may cause a reduced perception of vitality and mental health. Most effects had occurred within three months of starting carnitine supplementation.

In a similar trial,[27] recruits were taken from those who had at least two symptoms of carnitine deficiency and would therefore gain most from carnitine supplementation. These symptoms included muscle-cramping, lack of energy, muscle weakness, cardiomyopathy or no response to erythropoietin. The double-blind, placebo-controlled trial had a complete crossover design, with a wash-out period of six weeks between the test and placebo periods, which lasted 12 weeks each. Intravenous carnitine 20 mg/kg after each dialysis session for this duration was not found to have a significant benefit on quality of life in these chronic HD patients. The main complaint of lack of energy was unchanged as a result of the therapy and subjects did not notice any considerable improvements with the carnitine supplementation.

Although it may be too soon to recommend routine carnitine therapy for all HD patients, when there is an unexplained low response to rHuEPO, carnitine may be worth considering.[28] Large-scale clinical studies are required to provide unequivocal results, as well as optimal dose and duration, but there certainly seems to be a role for carnitine in some patients on dialysis, especially the elderly and those with cardiac disease.

## Heart disease

Carnitine is found in high concentrations in heart muscle, where it has important functions, including preventing lactic acid formation, which is damaging to the myocardium. The increasing amount of research in this area, including many clinical trials, points to the beneficial use of this supplement for many heart conditions. It has been shown that there is a reduction of up to 50% of both free and total carnitine in the failing heart.[29]

### *Cardiogenic shock*

Cardiogenic shock is a state of severe tissue hypoperfusion resulting from underlying pump dysfunction.[30] Cardiogenic shock usually starts as circulatory changes, which are followed by metabolic changes, leading to heart incompetence. After cardiogenic shock, autopsy has shown damage to more than 40% of the left ventricle. In a pilot study, carnitine was administered to 27 patients in addition to their usual medication. An intravenous bolus of 4 g was given initially, followed by a continuous infusion of 6 g/day for the duration of the cardiogenic shock conditions. Results showed that those patients given carnitine had an improvement in the condition, with a marked increase in survival time. Whereas the survival rate after cardiogenic shock is usually between 25% and 30%, over a ten-day period in the intensive care unit the patients given carnitine showed a survival rate of 78%. Carnitine may have protected against enzyme destruction and reduced cellular oxidative damage. An alternative explanation is that enhanced glucose utilisation may have decreased the hypoglycaemia which increases mortality in cardiogenic shock (see below under 'Insulin resistance').

### *Angina and congestive heart failure*

During myocardial ischaemia, when blood flow to the heart is reduced, carnitine levels in myocardial muscle decrease. Initially, there is a reduction in free carnitine and an increase in long-chain acyl carnitine, but if ischaemia continues, total carnitine also decreases by as much as 40%.[31] This results in an increase of free FAs and their metabolites within the cell cytoplasm, and a reduction of the oxidative processes necessary for energy production.[32] Supplementation with carnitine may therefore be of use in patients with ischaemic heart disease.

In one study,[32] 200 patients between the ages of 40 and 65 were recruited suffering from exercise-induced stable angina with classical onset and improvement with rest or after the use of sublingual glyceryl trinitrate. Half of the patients were treated with 2 g/day carnitine orally for six months, added to their normal therapy. The control patients continued as before, on their usual medication. Medication being used by the patients included nitro-compounds, calcium channel blockers, beta-blockers, antihypertensives, diuretics, cardiac glycosides, antiarrhythmics, anticoagulants and hypolipidaemics. Heart measurements, including heart rate, blood pressure, electrocardiogram (ECG), and cycle-exercise testing were performed for both groups of patients, as well as blood analysis. Results for the carnitine group showed significant and progressive improvements in cardiac function and quality of life. Although there were no differences in glycaemia or high-density lipoprotein cholesterol (HDL-C) for either group, there was a small but significant decrease in total cholesterol and triglycerides in the carnitine group. There was also a significant reduction of cardioactive drug consumption in the carnitine group, as seen in Table 6.1.

These results indicate that carnitine may be of importance in the control of exercise-induced stable angina, either alone or in combination with other heart medication.

In the year following myocardial infarction, patients are prone to cardiac complications, which often result in death. A trial was carried out to determine whether carnitine would have a protective effect on these patients.[33] One hundred and sixty patients who had suffered recent

**Table 6.1** Percentage decreases in heart medication seen in patients taking carnitine supplementation

| *Medication* | *% decrease* |
|---|---|
| Nitroglycerides | 60 |
| Other nitro-derivatives | 40 |
| Nifedipine | 33 |
| Diltiazem | 47 |
| Beta-blockers | 36 |
| Antihypertensives | 44 |
| Cardiac glycosides | 35 |
| Diuretics | 34 |
| Anticoagulants | 44 |
| Antiarrythmics | 70 |
| Hypolipidaemics | 61 |

acute myocardial infarction were included in the study. On discharge from hospital, the patients were randomly assigned to groups A or B. Group A received 2 g carnitine twice daily, for one year, in addition to the standard cardioactive medication. Group B acted as the control, receiving no carnitine supplementation. Throughout the study, at set intervals, heart measurements were carried out. Positive results were seen in group A in terms of cardiac events and life expectancy with significant differences for nearly all the parameters studied. Particularly striking were the differences in mortality of 1.2% in the carnitine group (one death caused by thromboembolism) and 12.5% in the control group (reinfarction and sudden death in eight cases and two extra-cardiac deaths). This study clearly showed that the addition of carnitine at a dose of 2 g twice daily to the usual heart medication, improved both quality of life and life expectancy in the year following myocardial infarction.

In a similar study involving 101 patients with suspected acute myocardial infarction, 2 g carnitine daily in three divided doses was compared with placebo. Since cardiac events after acute myocardial infarction are so rapid, treatment must be given promptly to avoid lasting damage to the heart. In this study carnitine was given within 10 hours of the onset of symptoms. After 28 days of treatment, the mean infarct size was significantly reduced in the carnitine group, as were cardiac events, including angina pectoris, left ventricular failure and arrhythmias. No side-effects were noted but the use of other heart medication was reduced in the carnitine group.[31]

Carnitine has also been used to shorten recovery time in children with heart failure. Twenty-four out of 91 children suffering from heart failure were given supplemental carnitine, at a dose of 50 mg/kg/day for 15 days. The children in the test group showed a marked improvement over the controls and decreased recovery time.[34]

One recent, small study ($n$ = 30) reported that there was a parallel correlation between plasma and urinary carnitine levels and altered left ventricular function, which occurs secondary to congestive heart failure, and therefore this could act as a marker for the disease.[35] The authors suggest that these increased levels may be due to leakage of carnitine from cardiac tissue or due to a defect in carnitine transport mechanisms.

In view of these and many other reports, which have been reviewed elsewhere,[3] the role of carnitine in heart disease seems promising. The reduction in mortality in post-myocardial infarction patients is very encouraging, as are the many other significant improvements to cardiac parameters seen with carnitine supplementation.

## Insulin resistance

The role of carnitine in glucose metabolism and insulin deficiency has been studied.[11] Twenty-five volunteers were recruited who had no metabolic disorders or problems of the liver, kidneys or heart muscle. In the first phase of the study, the subjects were given an infusion of 5% glucose over 2 hours, after which blood samples were taken. In the second part of the trial, the same subjects received the glucose infusion which had 2 g carnitine added to it. Hence the same subjects were acting as the test subjects and the controls. The addition of carnitine reduced insulin secretion but blood sugar levels were still decreased and remained at normal levels, resulting in an overall improvement in glucose metabolism. This may be relevant in situations where enhanced glucose utilisation is required through non-insulin pathways, such as in the period following myocardial infarction, when a reduction in insulin secretion usually leads to hypoglycaemia that increases mortality in heart failure and cardiogenic shock.

Reduced sensitivity to the hypoglycaemic effect of insulin is also a problem in chronic renal failure. This may be due to uraemic toxins, vitamin D deficiency and anaemia. A small trial was carried out using 13 HD patients, none of whom had a history of diabetes. It was found that carnitine improved insulin sensitivity in these patients, possibly by regulating the cell energy metabolism or by reducing free FAs.[36] Moreover, carnitine has been recommended in a list of nutritional strategies that may be of benefit to diabetic patients due to this effect.[37] Larger studies are required to confirm these findings.

### Alzheimer's disease

An ester form of carnitine, acetyl L-carnitine, is found with free plasma carnitine and other acyl esters.[38] This form of carnitine has been used as a neuroprotective agent in Alzheimer's disease and other dementias, as it crosses the blood–brain barrier when administered by both oral and intravenous routes. In several clinical trials,[39] acetyl L-carnitine improved cognitive and behavioural functions at doses of between 1.5 and 3 g daily, in both short-term (three months) and long-term (one-year) studies. In all trials, safety and tolerability were good. Acetyl carnitine seems to be a promising agent in neurological disease including Alzheimer's disease and also in ageing, stroke and diabetic neuropathy, with any side-effects, particularly of the gastrointestinal tract, being infrequent and transient.[38] However, in a recent one-year multicentre, double-blind, placebo-controlled, randomised trial of acetyl L-carnitine in early onset Alzheimer's disease there was no significant difference in decline between the treated and the control subjects.[40] Further clinical trials of long duration are therefore warranted to determine if indeed acetyl carnitine would be beneficial in Alzheimer's disease.

### Rett syndrome

Carnitine has also been investigated in Rett syndrome. This is a neurological disorder that affects girls and that involves the progressive loss of intellectual and motor skills, resulting in severe mental retardation. A randomised, placebo-controlled, double-blind trial was carried out in 35 Rett syndrome patients. The subjects were treated with carnitine (100 mg/kg/day) or placebo for eight weeks in a crossover design, with a wash-out period of eight weeks in between the two phases of the study. Parents (who were blinded to the study) reported an improvement of the condition while on carnitine. These improvements included improved eye contact and concentration, lack of daytime sleepiness, improved vocalisation and increased mobility. However, due to the side-effect of diarrhoea experienced by some subjects and a fishy body or urine odour reported by others, the carnitine period was identified by the parents, which may have affected results. Also the short duration of the trial did not uncover any long-term benefits (or drawbacks) to carnitine supplementation in these patients.[41]

## Human immunodeficiency virus (HIV)

A group of researchers have found that carnitine is beneficial in patients with the human immunodeficiency virus (HIV).[42] The patients received 6 g carnitine daily for six months, which led to a decrease in lymphocyte breakdown. Subsequent *in vitro* studies by the same research group suggested that carnitine acts on the immune system, rather than directly on the virus and may be of use in combination with anti-viral drugs. Other studies have found that carnitine and acetyl L-carnitine can correct the secondary carnitine deficiency in HIV patients, which may be due to malabsorption, kidney problems (leading to increased renal excretion), antibiotics and anti-viral medication and the loss of adipose tissue resulting in altered fatty acid metabolism.[38,43]

## Beta-thalassaemia major

Carnitine has also been given with promising results to transfusion-dependent β-thalassaemia major patients, who suffer from a genetic abnormality in which there is continued production of fetal haemoglobin resulting in clinical symptoms of haemolytic anaemia. The administration of oral carnitine led to an increased interval between transfusions.[44]

## Other uses

Other indications for carnitine therapy include anorexia, diphtheria and male infertility.[3] To date the evidence for all of these uses is not conclusive and studies in these areas have been small scale. It has been suggested that the muscle weakness and generalised fatigue associated with chronic fatigue symptom is also associated with carnitine deficiency. Some clinical trials have shown that periods of muscle weakness are related to low carnitine levels, which can be corrected with carnitine supplementation, but other studies have shown less promising results.[38,45] Several clinical trials have also shown that 2–3 g carnitine daily may be helpful in long-term weight loss for obese people, which usually involves low-calorie diets and physical exercise, both of which have a tendency to reduce carnitine levels.[4] Large-scale controlled trials are necessary to determine the clinical relevance of these findings.

## Drug interactions

### Valproic acid

It has been known for several years that anticonvulsant drugs, whether taken alone or in combination regimens, cause a decrease in total and/or free carnitine levels.[46] Initial studies were undertaken when it was noticed that side-effects of valproic acid, such as oedema, failure to thrive, thrombocytopenia, leukopenia and a Reye-like syndrome, were very similar to the symptoms of carnitine deficiency. Valproic acid is widely used as an antiepileptic agent in both adults and children and although generally well tolerated, it has been associated with fatal hepatotoxicity in 1 out of 49 000 adults and 1 out of 800 children below the age of two years.[47]

In one study it was found that plasma total and free carnitine levels were significantly reduced in 14 severely handicapped patients treated with valproic acid, compared with patients receiving other anticonvulsant therapy, and 27 healthy control subjects.[46] However, the patients with low carnitine levels did not show clinical symptoms of carnitine deficiency, which are difficult to assess in handicapped patients. All subjects received the same diet to eliminate carnitine dietary differences. There was an inverse relationship between the dose of valproic acid administered and the carnitine levels. The 14 valproic acid patients were then treated with 50 mg/kg of carnitine daily for four weeks and the carnitine levels returned to normal.

In another, larger study using 471 patients from a children's hospital, every serum sample submitted for anticonvulsant drug levels was also measured for total carnitine, free carnitine and carnitine ester levels, over ten months. The patients included in the study were receiving phenobarbital, valproic acid, phenytoin, carbamazepine, ethosuximide, primidone and methylphenobarbital. Control carnitine levels were taken from the serum samples of 32 healthy children. It was found that carnitine levels were affected in 23% of patients taking valproate, and also in 36% of patients taking phenobarbital, 12% of those taking phenytoin, and 8% of those taking carbamazepine.[48] A drawback to this study was that baseline values (before anticonvulsant therapy) were not taken, so it is not definite that the reduced levels were entirely due to the antiepileptic therapy.

Although other antiepileptic therapy has also been associated with reduced carnitine levels, as shown by this study, long-term valproate therapy has been particularly correlated with reduced concentrations of carnitine, especially in children. This correlation has been well reviewed in the literature[47] and several mechanisms have been suggested. These include the formation of valproyl CoA and valproylcarnitine, leading to competition of carnitine uptake, the formation of valproic acid metabolites that inhibit β-oxidation, and the resulting decrease in cell energy. A panel of nine paediatric neurologists has reviewed much of the recent work in this area and concluded that the valproate toxicity was indeed related to a reduction of carnitine. In 1996 they met to issue guidelines on the supplementation of carnitine in epilepsy.[12] Clinically, this work is very important, as valproate toxicity is associated with hepatotoxicity and can be fatal, especially in infants. Intravenous, high-dose carnitine therapy may be life saving in some cases, where there is hepatotoxicity due to either valproate overdose or a secondary carnitine deficiency. However, it is interesting to note that valproate-induced toxicity is not always due to carnitine deficiency, as was demonstrated in a case of a three-year-old girl who died from hepatic failure while receiving valproic acid, despite carnitine supplementation.[49] Nevertheless, there is a strong recommendation for oral carnitine supplementation in valproate patients, especially those less than two years of age who are receiving multiple anticonvulsant therapy or those with renal disease or in other high risk groups for hepatotoxicity, such as failure to thrive, malnutrition and chronic illness. Recommended dosage is 100 mg/kg/day or 2 g/day, whichever is less.

### Isotretinoin

Musculoskeletal disturbances are often reported in patients receiving isotretinoin for acne, and can be severe enough to warrant the discontinuation of treatment. Because similar symptoms are also often reported in carnitine deficiency, carnitine supplementation was tested in isotretinoin patients. A group of 230 patients taking the retinoid were included in the study and 16% showed muscular symptoms after approximately two weeks. Half of these patients received carnitine supplementation and the remainder was the control group and received placebo. In the carnitine group symptoms disappeared after 5–6 days, whereas in the placebo group symptoms continued, resulting in two patients discontinuing treatment and a further four receiving analgesics.[50]

### Pivampicillin

Carnitine has also been studied in pivampicillin therapy. Pivampicillin has a pivalic acid moiety, which enhances the absorption of the antibiotic.

Pivalate forms an ester with carnitine, decreasing carnitine levels. Administration of exogenous carnitine in patients on pivampicillin therapy avoids this and prevents the side-effects which would result, including decreased energy metabolism.[51]

## Side-effects

In general, few side-effects are seen with carnitine. As stated above, diarrhoea can be a problem and other gastrointestinal effects have also been reported.[3] A fishy body or urine odour was noticed in some subjects.[41] In a few cases, neurological patients taking carnitine experienced agitation and aggression.[38] One patient in an HD study withdrew after two weeks of carnitine supplementation as he observed an increase in blood glucose and insulin requirement,[1] but this finding has not been confirmed in larger studies. In fact, carnitine improved insulin sensitivity in renal failure patients on HD,[36] as described above.

Patients treated with acetyl carnitine have reported agitation, nausea and vomiting and in some cases alcohol tolerance was altered. Taking acetyl carnitine with food was shown to reduce these symptoms.[38]

In spite of these minor side-effects, carnitine remains a safe supplement. However, DL-carnitine, which is a mixture of the two isomeric forms of carnitine and is often sold, should be avoided as the D-isomer can lead to toxic effects (as described above).

## Conclusions

Carnitine seems to be a semi-essential component of the human body, with many promising uses. Although primary deficiency is rare, depletion due to a secondary cause, whether as a side-effect of medication or as a result of another disease, can occur. The main uses of carnitine are in HD patients and in heart disease, but other effects of carnitine may also become clinically relevant as the research and evidence for this nutraceutical increase.

## References

1. Kletzmayr J, Mayer G, Legenstein E, *et al.* Anemia and carnitine supplementation in hemodialyzed patients. *Kidney Int* 1999; 55(suppl 69): S93–S106.
2. Li Wan Po A. Carnitine: a scientifically exciting molecule. *Pharm J* 1990; 245: 388–389.

3. Kelly G S. L-Carnitine: therapeutic applications of a conditionally essential amino acid. *Altern Med Rev* 1998; 3: 345–360.
4. Walter P, Schaffhauser A O. L-Carnitine, a 'vitamin-like substance' for functional food. Proceedings of the symposium on L-carnitine, April 28 to May 1, 2000, Zermatt, Switzerland. *Ann Nutr Metab* 2000; 44: 75–96.
5. Sulkers E J, Lafeber H N, Goudoever J B, *et al.* L-Carnitine. *Lancet* 1990; 335: 1215.
6. Rodriguez-Benitez P, Perez-Garcia R, Arenas J, *et al.* L-Carnitine in dialysis, more than a commercial affair. *Nephrol Dial Transplant* 2000; 15: 1477–1478.
7. Rebouche C J, Chenard C A. Metabolic fate of dietary carnitine in human adults: identification and quantification of urinary and fecal metabolites. *J Nutr* 1991; 121: 539–546.
8. Harper P, Elwin C E, Cdererbald G. Pharmacokinetics of intravenous and oral bolus doses of L-carnitine in healthy subjects. *Eur J Clin Pharmacol* 1988; 35: 555–562.
9. Anon. Carnitine deficiency. *Lancet* 1991; 335: 631–633.
10. Brass E P, Hiatt W R. The role of carnitine and carnitine supplementation during exercise in man and in individuals with special needs. *J Am Coll Nutr* 1998; 3: 207–215.
11. Grandi M, Perderzoli S, Sacchetti C. Effect of acute carnitine administration on glucose insulin metabolism in healthy subjects. *Int J Clin Pharmacol Res* 1997; 17: 143–147.
12. De Vivo D, Bohan T P, Coulter D L, *et al.* L-Carnitine supplementation in childhood epilepsy: current perspectives. *Epilepsia* 1998; 39: 1216–1225.
13. Etzioni A, Levy J, Nitzan M, *et al.* Systemic carnitine deficiency exacerbated by a strict vegetarian diet. *Arch Dis Child* 1984; 59: 177–179.
14. Shortland G J, Walter J H. L-Carnitine. *Lancet* 1990; 335: 1215.
15. Winter S C, Zorn E M, Vance W H. Carnitine deficiency. *Lancet* 1990; 335: 981–982.
16. Chalmers R A, Bain M D, Stacey T E, *et al.* Carnitine deficiency. *Lancet* 1990; 335: 982.
17. Alp H, Orbak Z, Akcay F, *et al.* Plasma and urine carnitine levels and carnitine supplemenation in children with malnutrition. *J Trop Pediatr* 1999; 45: 294–296.
18. Brass E P. Supplemental carnitine and exercise. *Am J Clin Nutr* 2000; 72(suppl): 618S–623S.
19. Crayhorn R. Carnitine may benefit athletes. *J Am Coll Nutr* 1998; 17: 649–652.
20. Kooistra M P, Struyvenberg A, van Es A. The response to recombinant human erythropoietin in patients with the anemia of end-stage renal disease is correlated with serum carnitine levels. *Nephron* 1991; 57: 127–128.
21. Matsumoto Y, Amano I, Hirose S, *et al.* Effects of L-carnitine supplementation on renal anemia in poor responders to erythropoietin. *Blood Purif* 2001; 19: 24–32.
22. Lilien M R, Duran M, Quak J M E, *et al.* Oral L-carnitine does not decrease erythropoietin requirement in pediatric dialysis. *Pediatr Nephrol* 2000; 15: 17–20.
23. Caruso U, Leone L, Cravotto E, *et al.* Effects of L-carnitine on anemia in aged

hemodialysis patients treated with recombinant human erythropoietin: a pilot study. *Dialysis Transplant* 1998; 27: 498–506.

24. Matsumoto Y, Sato M, Ohashi H, *et al.* Effects of L-carnitine supplementation on cardiac morbidity in hemodialyzed patients. *Am J Nephrol* 2000; 20: 201–207.
25. Sakurabayashi T, Takaesu Y, Haginoshita S, *et al.* Improvement of myocardial fatty acid metabolism through L-carnitine administration to chronic hemodialysis patients. *Am J Nephrol* 1999; 19: 480–484.
26. Sloan R, Kastan B, Rice S, *et al.* Quality of life during and between hemodialysis treatments: role of L-carnitine supplementation. *Am J Kidney Dis* 1998; 32: 265–272.
27. Semeniuk J, Shalansky K F, Taylor N, *et al.* Evaluation of the effect of intravenous L-carnitine on quality of life in chronic hemodialysis patients. *Clin Nephrol* 2000; 54: 470–477.
28. Bommer J. Saving erythropoietin by administering L-carnitine? *Nephrol Dial Transplant* 1999; 14: 2819–2821.
29. Sole M, Jeejeebhoy K N. Conditioned nutritional requirements and the pathogenesis and treatment of myocardial failure. *Curr Opin Clin Nutr Metab Care* 2000; 3: 417–424.
30. Corbucci G G, Loche F. L-Carnitine in cardiogenic shock therapy: pharmacodynamic aspects and clinical data. *Int J Clin Pharmacol Res* 1993; 13: 87–91.
31. Singh R B, Niaz M A, Agaewal P, *et al.* A randomised, double-blind, placebo-controlled trial of L-carnitine in suspected acute myocardial infarction. *Postgrad Med J* 1996; 72: 45–50.
32. Cacciatore L, Cerio R, Ciarimboli M, *et al.* The therapeutic effect of L-carnitine in patients with exercise-induced stable angina: a controlled study. *Drugs Exp Clin Res* 1991; 17: 225–335.
33. Davini P, Bigalli A, Lamanna F, *et al.* Controlled study on L-carnitine therapeutic efficacy in post-infarction. *Drugs Exp Clin Res* 1992; 18: 355–365.
34. Ergur A T, Tanzer F, Cetinkaya O. Serum-free carnitine levels in children with heart failure. *J Trop Pediatr* 1999; 45: 168–169.
35. El-Aroussy W, Rizk A, Mayhoub G, *et al.* Plasma carnitine levels as a marker of impaired left ventricular functions. *Mol Cell Biochem* 2000; 213: 37–41.
36. Gunal A I, Celiker H, Donder E, *et al.* The effect of L-carnitine on insulin resistance in hemodialysed patients with chronic renal failure. *J Nephrol* 1999; 12: 38–40.
37. McCarty M F. Toward a wholly nutritional therapy for type 2 diabetes. *Med Hypotheses* 2000; 54: 483–487.
38. Furlong J H. Acetyl-L-carnitine: metabolism and applications in clinical practice. *Altern Med Rev* 1996; 1: 85–93.
39. Calvani M, Carta A, Caruso G, *et al.* Action of acetyl-L-carnitine in neurodegeneration and Alzheimer's disease. *Ann NY Acad Sci* 1992; 663: 483–486.
40. Thal L J, Calvani M, Amato A, *et al.* A 1-year controlled trial of acetyl-L-carnitine in early-onset AD. *Neurology* 2000; 55: 811–815.
41. Ellaway C, Williams K, Leonard H, *et al.* Rett syndrome: randomised controlled trial of L-carnitine. *J Child Neurol* 1999; 14: 162–167.
42. Famularo G, De Simone C, Cifone G. Carnitine stands on its own in HIV treatment. *Arch Intern Med* 1999; 159: 1143.

43. Patrick L. Nutrients and HIV: part three – *N*-acetylcysteine, alpha-lipoic acid, L-glutamine, and L-carnitine. *Altern Med Rev* 2000; 5: 290–305.
44. Yesilipek M A, Hazar V, Yegin O. L-Carnitine treatment in beta thalassemia major. *Acta Haematol* 1998; 100: 162–163.
45. Werbach M R. Nutritional strategies for treating chronic fatigue syndrome. *Altern Med Rev* 2000; 5: 93–108.
46. Ohtani Y, Endo F, Matsuda I. Carnitine deficiency and hyperammonemia associated with valproic acid therapy. *J Pediatr* 1982; 101: 782–785.
47. Raskind J Y, El-Chaar G M. The role of carnitine supplementation during valproic acid therapy. *Ann Pharmacother* 2000; 34: 630–638.
48. Hug G, McGraw C, Bates S, *et al.* Reduction of serum carnitine concentrations during anticonvulsant therapy with phenobarbital, valproic acid, phenytoin, and carbamazepine in children. *J Pediatr* 1991; 119: 799–802.
49. Laub M C, Paetzke-Brunner I, Jaeger G. Serum carnitine during valproic acid therapy. *Epilepsia* 1986; 27: 559–562.
50. Georgala S, Schulpis K, Georgala C, *et al.* L-Carnitine supplementation in patients with cystic acne on isotretinoin therapy. *J Eur Acad Dermatol Venereol* 1999; 13: 205–209.
51. Melegh B, Pap M, Molnar D, *et al.* Carnitine administration ameliorates the changes in energy metabolism caused by short-term pivampicillin medication. *Eur J Pediatr* 1997; 156: 795–799.

# 7

# Flaxseed and flaxseed oil

Flaxseed (*Linum usitatissimum*), also known as linseed, has been used traditionally for its fibre, which was woven to make cloth, and its seeds, which provided oil for food and paint.[1] Early writings also describe the use of both seeds and oil to treat various medical conditions.[2] Over the last ten years or so, flaxseed has been 'rediscovered' and its benefits to health are again being sought. Many animal and human studies have been carried out on the role of flaxseed in the prevention and treatment of many diseases, including heart disease, hypertension, inflammatory and autoimmune disease and cancer.

## Properties and structure

### Essential fatty acids

The fatty acid (FA) component of flaxseed oil contains more than 50% α-linoleic acid (ALA), which is an essential fatty acid. There are many sources of ALA, of which flaxseed is the richest[1] (Table 7.1).

Most FAs can either come from food or be synthesised in the body, but essential FAs cannot be made by the body and must therefore be ingested. There are two essential FAs necessary to humans: ALA and linoleic acid. In ALA there are 18 carbon atoms with three unsaturated bonds, starting at the third carbon atom, and it is sometimes referred to as a polyunsaturated fatty acid (PUFA) or superunsaturated FA. It is also known as an omega-3 (ω3 or n3) FA, denoting the position of the carbon atom at which the first double bond starts. Linoleic acid is also polyunsaturated, with the first double bond at the sixth carbon atom. It is therefore known as an ω6 FA. ALA can be written as 18 : 3ω3 (18 carbon atoms, 3 double bonds, 1st double bond at carbon 3 from the methyl end) and linoleic acid can be written as 18 : 2ω6 (18 carbon atoms, 2 double bonds, 1st double bond at carbon 6 from the methyl end) (Figure 7.1).[1,3]

Saturated FAs have no double bonds and are found in all food fats and oils, but predominantly in hard fats, such as animal fats. An excess

**Table 7.1** Sources of α-linoleic acid (ALA)[1]

| *Source of oil* | *Percentage of fatty acids as ALA* |
|---|---|
| Flaxseed | 50% |
| Candlenut | 30% |
| Hemp seed | 20% |
| Pumpkin seed | 0–15% |
| Canola | 0–10% |
| Walnut | 3–11% |
| Soybean | 5–7% |

of saturated FAs can lead to coronary problems. However, recommendations to replace saturated FAs with unsaturated FAs in order to improve coronary health have resulted in replacement by ω6 rather than ω3 PUFAs. This has led to the modern, western diet including far more ω6 FAs than ω3, in a ratio of approximately 20–30 : 1, although ideally the ratio should be almost equal. Moreover, fish consumption, which was a source of ω3 oils, has decreased in recent years. Also, due to modern food industry and agricultural methods, with an emphasis on production, the ω3 content of many foods, including meat, fish, eggs and vegetables is much lower than formerly. As a result many people are deficient in the ω3 essential FA ALA.[3]

Both ω6 and ω3 FAs are precursors of longer chain eicosanoids, such as prostaglandins, thromboxanes and leukotrienes. Those derived from ω6 FAs have opposing properties to those derived from ω3 and therefore a balance is required. A diet rich in ω6 and lacking in ω3 tends

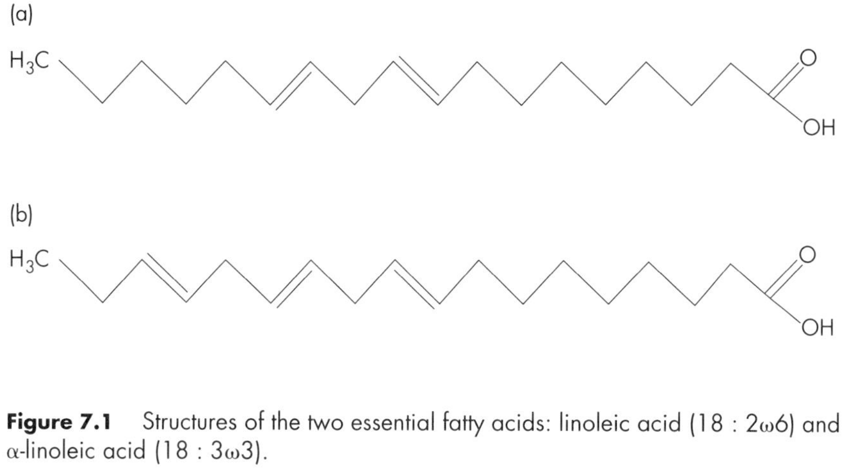

(a)

(b)

**Figure 7.1** Structures of the two essential fatty acids: linoleic acid (18 : 2ω6) and α-linoleic acid (18 : 3ω3).

to lead to thrombi, blood aggregation and cardiovascular disease, as well as allergies, inflammation and diabetes. Fish oils have long been recognised as a source of long-chain ω3 PUFAs, and many researchers have studied these oils. However, flaxseed provides the richest plant source precursor, ALA, which is converted to these long-chain FAs, and provides a way to correct deficiency and prevent diseases associated with decreased ω3 FAs. Only recently have the benefits of flaxseed as a source of these essential FAs been realised.

One advantage of ALA over fish oils is that the problem of insufficient intake of vitamin E does not occur when plant sources are used.[3] Moreover, as well as being a precursor for longer chain ω3 FAs, ALA has clinically relevant effects in its own right, which offers another benefit over ω3-containing fish oils.[4]

## Oil or seed?

In a crossover study,[2] flaxseed oil capsules were taken three times daily (20 g oil per day, containing 12 g ALA) and compared with flaxseed flour which was added to breakfast cereal, soup or yoghurt (50 g flour per day, containing 12 g ALA). The subjects were five young, healthy women and there was a wash-out period of two weeks between the two four-week periods. Venous blood samples were obtained for FA analysis. The bioavailability of the ALA was similar in each case, resulting in lowered blood lipids. Also, although flaxseed is a calorific food (280 kcal/50 g), over the four-week period there was no weight gain in the subjects, indicating that other energy sources had been displaced from the diet.

In another experiment by the same team of researchers,[2] flaxseed flour sprinkled on foods was compared with bread made from the flour, both providing 50 g/day of flaxseed for four weeks. Fatty acid profiles of the nine subjects did not differ significantly between the two groups, with the effect being mainly on the low-density lipoprotein cholesterol (LDL-C). Again no weight gain was reported. Caution is required before conclusions are reached from such a small number of subjects, especially since all the subjects were young and healthy. However, from these experiments it follows that the form in which flaxseed is consumed, whether flour, oil or in baked goods, does not seem to affect the bioavailability of the ALA.

The optimum amount of ALA is about one or two teaspoonfuls of the oil daily (2–9 g).[1] While still in the seed, the oil can keep for years, but once extracted it should be stored carefully and shelf-dated, as it is sensitive to heat and light. Freezing is an alternative way of ensuring that the oil is in prime condition while being stored. Moreover, plant oils are often hydrogenated during processing, which destroys the ALA found in the pure oil. It is therefore important to ensure that flaxseed oil purchased for its therapeutic properties is not in this form.[5]

## Uses of flaxseed and flaxseed oil

### Cardiac events and atherosclerosis

As already described, the eicosanoids from arachidonic acid, which are produced from ω6 FAs, are hyperlipidaemic, prothrombotic and proaggregatory and lead to atherosclerotic disease if present in too high a concentration. The eicosanoids from ω3 FAs, however, have the opposite effects.[3] Flaxseed would therefore seem a good supplement for lowering cholesterol and improving heart function.

In a large trial carried out in 1994[6] the effect of an ALA-rich, 'Mediterranean' diet was compared with a usual diet in the survivors of a first myocardial infarction (MI). The MI survivors were randomly assigned to the experimental diet ($n$ = 302), or continued with their normal diets ($n$ = 303). The experimental diet included a high intake of ALA, and more bread, root vegetables, green vegetables and fruit. They were also advised to eat more fish, less meat and replace butter and cream with margarine supplied by the study, which was canola oil (rapeseed oil)-based and provided about 5% ALA. Any subject with a condition that might limit survival was excluded, as well as those with advanced heart failure, hypertension (>180/110), and those unable to complete an exercise test. A reduction of coronary events and cardiac deaths of close to 70% was seen in the experimental group over five years. There were 20 deaths in the control group, 16 of which were due to cardiac causes and eight of which were sudden. In the experimental group there were only eight deaths, three from cardiac causes and none were sudden. The high intake of fruits and vegetables in the experimental group led to a significantly higher concentration of antioxidants in the plasma when measured at 52 weeks. Although these may well have increased the positive effects of the experimental diet, it was concluded that the increase in ALA in the diet also seemed to have significant consequences for coronary health.

*Flaxseed or fish oils?*

Due to the health benefits of ω3 FAs over ω6 oils, research has been carried out to see if the flaxseed plant source has the same advantages as marine sources on lipoprotein metabolism. Evaluation of many human studies,[7] led to the conclusion that ALA was equivalent to ω6 fish oils and not as beneficial as ω3 fish oils in its effects on lowering serum cholesterol, unless ingested in very large quantities (60 ml oil). This is because long-chain ω3 FA production from ALA depends on the amount of ω6 FA already present. Fish oils provide long-chain ω3 PUFAs, eicosapentaenoic acid (EPA, 20 : 5ω3) and docosahexaenoic acid (DHA, 22 : 6ω3), whereas flaxseed provides an ω3 precursor, which must be converted to these beneficial long-chain ω3 PUFAs. Since most people have a vast excess of ω6 FAs, the ω6 pathways are preferred and long-chain ω6 FAs are produced (18 : 2ω6⇒20 : 4ω6). The conversion of the ω3 precursor to the long-chain FAs from ALA is therefore more significant over a long time period of time, or with very large intakes.

In a controlled, randomised, double-blind, crossover study,[8] the effect of low-dose flaxseed or fish oils on subjects ($n = 26$) consuming diets with a high or low polyunsaturated/saturated FA content was investigated. All subjects took olive oil capsules (consisting mostly of oleic acid, 18 : 1ω9) for three months as a placebo. They were then randomly assigned to take flaxseed oil (35 mg of ALA daily) or fish oil (35 mg of EPA daily) in capsules for three months, before crossing over to the other supplement. Blood samples and diet records were taken every three months. Neither flaxseed oil nor fish oil capsules significantly altered plasma total cholesterol, LDL-C and HDL-C. However, it was found that fish oil reduced plasma triacylglycerides in the low polyunsaturated/saturated group, which is the diet favoured in modern, western societies. Plasma triacyglycerol, as well as LDL and total cholesterol levels may be a predictor of coronary heart disease. This effect, however, was not seen in the flaxseed oil subjects and this may have been due to the small dose used.

In a small trial, 11 healthy, young, non-smoking males were randomly assigned to take either 40 g of flaxseed oil (containing over 55% ω3) or 40 g of sunflower seed oil (containing over 55% ω6) for 23 days, in addition to a low-fat diet.[9] Blood samples were taken on day 1 and day 23 and the blood platelet FAs were analysed. FA ω6 : ω3 ratios varied from 1 : 2 in the flaxseed group to 30 : 1 in the sunflower group. The long-chain ω3 PUFA EPA more than doubled in the study time in the flaxseed group. This indicated that flaxseed oil is indeed a good precursor for EPA, which is associated with decreased collagen-induced platelet aggregation and thrombosis. No conclusions were reached as to the optimal ratios of ω6 : ω3 in the diet or to the exact mechanism of action of decreased aggregation.

### *Aortic compliance*

Obesity is one of the main risk factors for coronary heart disease (CHD). Another risk factor is aortic compliance, or elasticity, which is related to arterial function. A decrease in aortic compliance occurs with advancing age, hypertension, diabetes and atherosclerosis. Fish oil supplementation has been shown to improve aortic compliance and therefore an experiment was carried out to determine if ALA from flaxseed would also have a positive effect on this parameter.[10] Fifteen middle-aged, obese subjects were entered into the study, which involved four diets for four weeks each (two intervention periods with a control at each end): saturated FA/high fat, flaxseed oil/low fat, sunola oil (oleic acid-rich sunflower oil)/low fat and saturated FA/high fat. It was found that supplementation with 20 g of flaxseed oil daily, improved aortic compliance with a resulting improvement in arterial function over the four-week study. This finding may have significant effects in elderly, diabetic or obese patients, all of whom show a tendency towards decreased aortic elasticity.

### *Cholesterol-lowering effects*

Ten healthy, young adults were involved in another small experiment, which used a randomised, crossover design.[11] Two control muffins containing no flaxseed but providing 1.4 g ALA daily from canola oil, or two flaxseed muffins containing 25 g flaxseed per muffin and providing 9 g ALA daily, were eaten for four weeks and then the groups were crossed over. Blood samples were taken for the analysis of blood lipoproteins. After two weeks of flaxseed muffins, plasma concentrations of long-chain ω3 had increased, as expected. Total cholesterol and LDL-C had decreased significantly by 6% and 9% respectively, and these values remained low for the duration of the control four weeks. At week 4, total cholesterol and LDL-C were similar in the two groups. However, plasma HDL-C and total cholesterol were unchanged in both groups. The authors questioned whether the decrease in LDL-C may be attributed to the increased excretion of bile salts, as a result of the laxative effect of the flaxseed oil in the flaxseed muffin group.

In an animal experiment, 30 rabbits were divided into four different diet groups, as shown in Table 7.2, and were used in an experiment to determine the effect of flaxseed on hypercholesterol-induced atherosclerosis.[12] Atherosclerotic plaques on the aorta were detected and expressed as a percentage of luminal surface. Atherosclerotic plaques were not seen in groups 1 and 2, but in group 3 the aorta was almost covered with plaque. In group 4, the addition of flaxseed to the cholesterol diet was shown to reduce hypercholesterolaemic atherosclerosis by 46%, although total serum cholesterol and LDL-C were increased.

This led the researchers to consider whether the anti-atherosclerotic properties of flaxseed were possibly due to the lignans present in flaxseed rather than the ALA alone. As well as having a high concentration of ALA, flaxseed is also a rich source of plant lignans. Lignans are one of the classes of phytoestrogens and have many beneficial properties, including antioxidant properties, which may have a role in the prevention of CHD. To test this hypothesis, another experiment was carried out using another type of flaxseed, which has only 2–3% of its oil as ALA, but similar lignan content. Again, rabbits were used to determine the effect of the diets used in the previous experiment on cholesterol-induced atherosclerosis, but the low-ALA flaxseed was used.[13] The development of aortal atherosclerotic plaques was reduced by 69% in these rabbits, without significant changes in serum lipids. This experiment indeed seems to indicate that the lignan parts rather than ALA are responsible for these effects.

Similarly in a small-scale human trial,[14] the effect of partially defatted flaxseed (low ALA) was investigated in hyperlipidaemic men and women. Only postmenopausal women were included, and any subject with diabetes, liver disease or renal disease was excluded. Twenty-nine subjects (22 men, 7 women) completed the trial. The subjects ate four control muffins (no flaxseed) or four test muffins (defatted flaxseed) daily, for two three-week periods in a randomised, crossover design. There was a two-week wash-out period between each test period. Serum

**Table 7.2** Experimental rabbit diets used in an experiment to determine the effect of flaxseed on hypercholesterol-induced atherosclerosis[12]

| *Group* | *Diet* |
|---|---|
| Group 1 | Rabbit chow – control |
| Group 2 | Flaxseed (7.5 g/kg) |
| Group 3 | 1% cholesterol in rabbit chow |
| Group 4 | 1% cholesterol + flaxseed |

samples were obtained and analysed for serum lipids. The defatted flaxseed reduced the serum concentrations of total cholesterol and LDL-C in similar amounts to those given full-fat flaxseed in previous experiments, quoted by the authors. However, there was no effect on serum lipoprotein. As well as the lignan effects there are also beneficial effects from the seed-coat gum of flaxseed, which may be responsible for the hypolipidaemic action. Additional trials are required in which all the components are isolated, to determine exactly which part of the flaxseed is contributing to these effects. It would also be useful if the industry used a standard for flaxseed preparations so that consumers would have an idea of how much of each particular component is present in any particular product.

### *Stroke*

A recent follow-up study over 14 years examined the relationship between ω3 FA intake from fish and the risk of stroke in 79 839 American women.[15] The study found that those women who ate fish more than once a month had a lower risk of total stroke. In the case of thrombotic stroke, the risk was significantly reduced by 48% amongst women who ate fish two to four times weekly. All values were corrected for age, smoking and other cardiovascular risk factors. Moreover, as fish consumption increased, the risk of stroke decreased. This relationship was more evident amongst women who did not take aspirin regularly, as the strong effect of aspirin on the risk of thrombotic infarction masks the relationship between ω3 FA intake and risk. Since it was the ω3 FA intake from the fish that led to these results, it would follow that flaxseed would have the same effects in people who do not eat fish, but clinical trials are required to confirm this theory.

## Conclusion

In conclusion, the papers reviewed strongly suggest that flaxseed could be a beneficial supplement in the prevention of hypercholesterolaemia-induced heart attacks and strokes. For this use it would seem that whole flaxseed is superior to the purified oil, since both the lignans and the seed-coat gum also have beneficial effects, although the exact mechanism has yet to be confirmed. Unfortunately, most of the trials using flaxseed to date have been small, and studies using larger populations, as well as people who are in high risk categories would be beneficial.

### Diabetes

In the standard glucose test, blood is tested at intervals following ingestion of the test substance after an overnight fast. Bread made from flaxseed flour was compared with white bread, and flaxseed mucilage mixed with glucose was compared with glucose alone, in such a blood glucose determination using six healthy volunteers.[12] Both flaxseed flour and flaxseed mucilage reduced the post-meal blood glucose by about 27% in each case.

In a similar experiment comparing glucose tolerance after consuming flaxseed muffins or white flour muffins for four weeks,[11] the 30-minute glucose concentration was significantly lower in the flaxseed group. These results indicate a possible hypoglycaemic use for flaxseed, and there could be a benefit from the incorporation of flaxseed into foods and snack products aimed at the diabetic population.

### Immune status and inflammation

Different dietary fats are known to have an effect on the immune system and inflammation. Conflicting results as to the effect of dietary fats on immunocompetence in animal models have been reported.[16] For example, ingestion of fish oils led to an increased occurrence of collagen-induced arthritis in rats, but a decrease in mice. A preliminary study on humans was carried out in 1991.[16] The small study used ten healthy, young men. After an initial two-week control period during which all subjects consumed a basal diet, five subjects continued with the basal diet for test period one, while the other five received the basal diet supplemented with flaxseed oil. After eight weeks, the groups were crossed over, for a further eight weeks, which comprised test period two. Blood samples were drawn at intervals throughout the two test periods, to test for different components, and saliva samples were also taken. Peripheral blood mononuclear cells were isolated from the blood samples and cultured with mitogens. These are agents which promote division of lymphocytes and hence were used to measure humoral immunity (immunity caused by the body's own fluids). At the end of the control period and each test period, cell-mediated immunity was also tested by the hypersensitivity response of each subject on injecting a diluted antigen into the forearm. The antigens used were tuberculin protein derivative, mumps, tetanus toxoid, candida, trichophyton, streptokinase (Streptase) and coccidioidin. It was found that the supplemented diet suppressed some of the cell-mediated immunity from T cells, and decreased the delayed hypersensitivity response to the seven antigens, but the results were not statistically significant, possibly due to the small number of subjects used. From the mitogen tests, it was found that humoral immunity from B cells was not suppressed. Moreover, concentrations of immunoglobulins in serum, helper cells, suppressor cells, total B and T cells, complement fractions $C_3$ and $C_4$ and salivary immunoglobulin A (IgA), which are all involved in the immune system, did not vary between the two diets. From this small experiment, flaxseed did seem to somewhat affect the immunocompetence in humans, but the effect was not very substantial. More research is necessary in this area; if flaxseed does lead to suppression of the immune system this may be of use in autoimmune disease. However, this is also a concern for healthy people using flaxseed for other indications, as long-term use could lead to suppression of the immune system, which would be an unwanted effect.

There are many mediators in the processes involved with inflammation. These include the eicosanoids: prostaglandins (PG), thromboxanes (TX) and leukotrienes (LT), which can be proinflammatory or anti-inflammatory and are released from activated leukocytes in the target area.[17] From Figure 7.2 it can be seen that there are two competing pathways in forming these mediators. In (A), arachidonic acid, formed from the ω6 EFA linoleic acid, is converted via the cyclooxygenase and 5-lipoxygenase enzymes to $PGE_2$, $TXA_2$ and $LTB_4$. These are all proinflammatory. $PGE_2$ causes pain and dilation, whilst $LTB_4$ activates neutrophils. The net result is the pain, redness and swelling of inflammation. Non-steroidal anti-inflammatory drugs (NSAIDs) reduce inflammation by blocking this pathway. An alternative pathway for the formation of these mediators is shown in (B). ALA is enzymatically converted to EPA (which can also be ingested as fish oils as described above), that in turn forms PGs and LTs using the same enzymes, cyclooxygenase and 5-lipoxygenase. However, the PGs and LTs formed from the ω3 pathways are non-inflammatory or anti-inflammatory. Therefore it has been suggested that an increase in ALA would lead to less inflammation, by preference of the ω3 pathways.

### *Autoimmune disease*

Systemic lupus erythematosus (SLE) is an autoimmune, vascular disease, which usually comprises early inflammatory and late atherosclerotic events. A small study using flaxseed has been carried out on eight patients with SLE, in whom the lupus was present as lupus nephritis

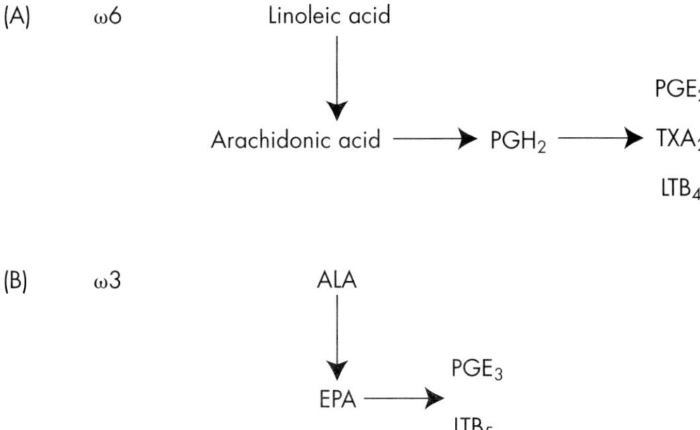


**Figure 7.2** Scheme showing the two pathways for the formation of prostaglandins (PG), leukotrienes (LT) and thromboxanes (TX). ALA, α-linoleic acid; EPA, eicosapentaenoic acid.

(affecting the kidney).[18] Flaxseed was chosen because it has been shown to have a role in atherosclerosis and in suppressing immunocompetence. Moreover, the lignan part of ALA has been shown to include strong platelet-activating factor (PAF) antagonists. PAF is involved in the initiation and propagation of the inflammation reaction, and in both animal and human lupus nephritis, PAF levels have been found to be elevated.[19] Therefore inhibition of PAF would be expected to reduce the inflammatory response.

The study[18] was composed of four stages as shown in Table 7.3. Flaxseed was found to improve renal function, measured by serum creatinine, creatinine clearance and urinary protein values. Throughout the flaxseed stages (I–III) there was PAF inhibition which was reversible and was not seen in stage IV, and inflammatory mechanisms improved. The flaxseed supplement at a dose of up to 30 g daily was well tolerated, but at the highest dose of 45 g daily, three patients suffered from diarrhoea. Total and LDL cholesterol were lowered in stages II and III and this effect continued throughout stage IV, even though the supplementation had been discontinued. These preliminary findings are interesting, but larger studies would be required to determine the clinical use of flaxseed in lupus nephritis. Since consuming 30 g of crushed flaxseed daily would not be palatable for some patients, some researchers have extracted large amounts of the lignan precursor from flaxseed.[20] This lignan precursor

**Table 7.3** The four stages of the study to show the effect of flaxseed on systemic lupus erythematosus (SLE)[18]

| *Stage* | *Duration* | *Dosage of flaxseed* |
|---|---|---|
| I | 4 weeks | 15 g daily |
| II | 4 weeks | 15 g twice daily |
| III | 4 weeks | 15 g three times daily |
| IV | 5 weeks | No supplementation |

showed renal protection similar to that provided by the whole flaxseed in animal models, and was well tolerated, but has not yet been used in human studies. (Additional trials in other kidney diseases are described below.)

Rheumatoid arthritis (RA) is an inflammatory disease that involves multiple synovial joints. RA patients show symptoms of inflammation, which include vasodilation, oedema, pain in movement and joint tenderness.[21] In a small trial, 30 g flaxseed oil daily was compared to 30 g safflower oil (ω6) daily for three months in 22 RA patients.[21] No clinical improvement in RA was seen in the flaxseed group compared with the safflower oil control group. It was expected that the ALA would decrease the arachidonic acid metabolites formed from ω6 FAs, which are proinflammatory and cause tissue destruction and pain, instead forming ω3 metabolites that are non-inflammatory, as described above. However, this did not seem to be the case. The authors suggest that three months of supplementation was not enough to alter the ω3 : ω6 ratio. Also zinc and other nutrients, such as vitamin E, are necessary to facilitate the conversion of ALA to its metabolites. Interestingly, these were found to be in low concentration in the RA patients.

Whereas the eicosanoids are responsible for the early symptoms of inflammatory disease, cytokines are involved in the late, destructive phase eventually leading to joint failure. The cytokines interleukin 1β (IL-1β) and tumour necrosis factor α (TNFα) increase inflammatory reactions and are also implicated in atherosclerosis.[22] Positive results using fish oil capsules as a source of EPA to decrease cytokine production have led researchers to investigate the effect of ALA from flaxseed as a precursor of these long-chain PUFAs. Twenty-eight healthy, young males completed an eight-week trial in which a sunflower oil diet was compared with a flaxseed oil diet (supplying approximately 14 g ALA daily). For the first four weeks, subjects ingested a sunflower oil diet or a flaxseed oil diet. For the following four weeks, they all continued with their respective diets, and all subjects also took nine fish oil capsules daily. Blood samples were withdrawn at weeks 0 (baseline), 4 and 8 and analysed for eicosanoids and cytokines. The results can be seen in Table 7.4, but it must be remembered that from week 4 to week 8 all subjects also took fish oil capsules.

ALA ingestion resulted in a decrease of TNFα and IL-1β by about 30%, and this decreased further to about 80% with the addition of fish oil. Although sunflower seed oil did not cause a change in the values of the cytokines, when fish oil was taken with sunflower oil (sunflower group, weeks 4–8) there was a marked decrease.[22] Although these results are based on healthy, young males, many other trials have been carried out using fish oils in RA patients. In a review of the use of fish oils in RA, the author concluded that the supplement should be taken for at least three or four months before reducing the dosage of NSAIDs.[23] Whether the same findings would apply to ALA remains to be seen, but certainly in theory ALA would be a good therapeutic tool, based on its ability to decrease production of TNFα and IL-1β. Indeed, many modern pharmacotherapies for RA are directed at the inhibition of these cytokines and flaxseed may have the same effect.

In summary, both immunocompetence and inflammation are cascade reactions involving many mediators. Flaxseed has been shown to affect some of these, resulting in immunosuppression and reduced inflammation. Whether these findings will lead to clinical use remains to be seen, but the evidence to date looks promising. Since treatment for these types of diseases is usually long-term, prolonged studies on large numbers of subjects are required before widespread use of flaxseed can be recommended.

**Table 7.4** Decreases in eicosanoids and cytokines as a result of flaxseed oil and sunflower oil

| | *Flaxseed group* | | *Sunflower seed group* | |
|---|---|---|---|---|
| | *Week 4* | *Week 8* | *Week 4* | *Week 8* |
| TNFα | 30% | 77% | ⇔ | 70% |
| IL-1β | 31% | 81% | ⇔ | 78% |
| $TXB_2$ | 29% | 48% | ⇔ | 52% |
| $PGE_2$ | 30% | 28% | ⇔ | 55% |

TNFα, tumour necrosis factor α; IL-1β, interleukin 1β; $TXB_2$, thromboxane $B_2$; $PGE_2$, prostaglandin $E_2$; ⇔, no change.

## Kidney disease

Kidney disease is often associated with inflammation, and the evidence showing an influence of flaxseed in reducing inflammation has led to investigations into the effect of flaxseed in kidney disease. In one such experiment, a rat model was used to determine the effect of flaxseed on polycystic kidney disease (PKD).[24] This condition involves progressive dilation of nephrons in young animals and inflammation and fibrosis with nephron loss in older animals. The rat model for this disease is useful, as it is very similar to the progression of the human disease. Forty-one rats were included and they were randomly assigned to receive either a normal (control) diet or a flaxseed-supplemented diet. After eight weeks, kidney tissue and serum were analysed. The flaxseed-fed rats showed a reduction in cystic change, less renal fibrosis and less macrophage infiltration, as well as lower serum creatinine levels. The authors suggest that flaxseed supplementation may be developed to treat chronic renal injury in humans.

## Women's health

As well as containing a high percentage of ALA, flaxseed is also a very good source of lignans, one of the main classes of phytoestrogens. These are non-steroidal compounds and are either of plant origin or derived from plant material once it has been ingested by the human body. The two classes of phytoestrogens are the lignans, which will be discussed here, and the isoflavones, for example genistein, found in legumes and beans, particularly soybeans. After consumption, enzymes in the gastrointestinal tract convert phytoestrogens to phenolic substances resembling the female hormone oestrogen. Hence the name phyto (= plant) oestrogens. The lignans formed from flaxseed precursors are enterodiol and enterolactone[25] and although many foods contain lignans, for example, cereals, fruits and vegetables, flaxseed is claimed to be the richest source.[26]

Epidemiologic data indicate that less than 25% of Japanese women, who have a diet high in soy products, suffer from hot flushes compared with 85% of North American women. These menopausal women also show a low incidence of hormone-related cancers and the incidence increases as diets become westernised. Since phytoestrogens show both weak oestrogenic activity and anti-oestrogenic effects, depending on the tissue and the concentration, research has been carried out in such areas as menopausal symptoms, breast cancer and osteoporosis.[27] In one study, flaxseed was shown to alter the menstrual cycle in premenopausal women.[28] In another study it was found that soy protein significantly reduced the frequency of hot flushes in a double-blind, multicentre, parallel, randomised, placebo-controlled trial involving 104 postmenopausal women.[29]

Once formed, lignans are circulated via the liver and excreted in the urine as glucuronide or sulfate conjugates.[26] Nine healthy, premenopausal women were included in a randomised, crossover trial to determine the dose–response of urinary lignan concentration to flaxseed intake, and additionally to assess whether raw and processed flaxseed would produce the same result.[25] The stage of the menstrual cycle was controlled in the experiment and subjects were not taking hormonal therapy or prescription medicines. A linear dose–response was seen as flaxseed ingestion increased from 5 g/day to 25 g/day. No plateau was seen at a dose of 25 g, indicating that further increases would lead to increased response. By the eighth day of ingestion, urinary and plasma lignans showed a significant, linear relationship, indicating that this is a good way of measuring plasma concentration. Although lignan metabolism showed variation among subjects, overall enterodiol was the lignan produced in the highest concentration. The second part of the experiment showed that processing did not affect the lignan production, as results from raw flaxseed and processed flaxseed (muffin or bread) were similar.

These results are promising for women in whom hormone replacement therapy (HRT) is contraindicated and for those who are worried about possible side-effects of HRT, as the lignans from flaxseed could have the same effects as exogenous oestrogen.

### Cancer

Urinary lignan excretion was found to be lower in breast cancer patients and higher in vegetarians, in whom there is a lower risk of cancer. Moreover, in certain populations in which there is a high consumption of isoflavones, particularly the Japanese who eat a lot of soy products, there was found to be a very low incidence of cancer. Therefore studies were carried out to investigate the effects of lignans on cancer, using animal models. Many researchers showed that lignans have hormonal action, and epidemiological studies have suggested that lignans have a protective effect against tumours, especially hormone-related cancers such as breast and prostate cancer, although direct evidence from human studies is lacking.[26]

To determine whether whole flaxseed, the lignans or the flaxseed oil (ALA) were responsible for its anti-tumour properties, a study using an isolated, purified lignan precursor (secoisolariciresinol-diglycoside, SD) as well as whole flaxseed and ALA was carried out on rats.[30] Supplementation was started 13 weeks after carcinogen administration, and whilst flaxseed oil and flaxseed both reduced the growth of existing mammary tumours, SD prevented the formation of new tumours. ALA acts by mechanisms other than through lignans and therefore the inhibition of cancer growth by flaxseed seems to be by various mechanisms, including properties of the oil and the lignans.

Other cancers have also been studied and it was found that lignans offer protection from cancer of the colon in rats and skin cancer in mice.[26] In an *in vitro* experiment on human colon tumour cells, it was found that the lignans reduced the proliferation of the cell lines.[31] In this case the lignans seem to be independent of oestrogenic activity and therefore the mechanism by which lignans inhibit tumours appears to be multifactorial, possibly related to antioxidant action.

### Constipation

In the crossover study mentioned above,[11] in which two flaxseed muffins or two white flour muffins were eaten daily for four weeks by a small group of young, healthy adults, bowel movements increased by 30% per week in the flaxseed period. This side-effect could possibly be used in the treatment of constipation, but no clinical trials were found for this use.

## Side-effects and contraindications

Flaxseed and flaxseed oil seem to be safe, with the main side-effect being diarrhoea.[11] In one controlled trial in which 22 patients took ALA to investigate its effect on RA, bleeding time was lengthened in the group ingesting ALA.[21] This suggests that patients receiving anticoagulation therapy, such as warfarin, should exercise caution while taking flaxseed, and regular blood tests would be advisable.

Several papers have been written on the possible benefits of ω3 FAs in pregnancy[32] and there also appear to be significant advantages for preterm infants,[33] although fish oil supplements have been used rather than flaxseed. During hormone-sensitive periods such as pregnancy and lactation, flaxseed may have adverse effects due to the effect of the lignans present. Such adverse effects have been found in animal studies[26] and so the risk must be weighed against possible benefits. Flaxseed supplements should not be recommended during pregnancy and lactation until conclusive evidence from human studies can prove that they are safe.

## Conclusions

In conclusion, flaxseed oil as well as the ground seeds seem to have promising value in the treatment of various chronic diseases, particularly in the prevention of cardiac events, and they may also offer protection against hormone-related cancers. This nutraceutical is easy to take, whether in the form of pure oil or added to foodstuffs in the course of a normal diet. A recent study found that enriching everyday foods, such as oil, margarine and salad dressing with ALA, and using flaxseed meal for food preparation (cakes, casseroles, sauces, etc.) leads to the desired health benefits without the necessity of long-term supplementation with encapsulated fish oils or an increase in fish consumption.[34] For those who prefer to take it as the oil or as ground seeds, the good safety profile and lack of interactions with other prescribed medicine make flaxseed an ideal supplement and the research indicates that adding ALA to the diet in any form would benefit many.

## References


1. Erasmus U. *Fats that Heal, Fats that Kill: the Complete Guide to Fats, Oils and Cholesterol*, 2nd edn. Burnaby BC, Canada: Alive Books, 1993.
2. Cunnane S C, Ganguli S, Menard C, *et al.* High α linoleic acid flaxseed (*Linum usitatissimum*): some nutritional properties in humans. *Br J Nutr* 1993; 69: 443–453.
3. Simopoulos A P. Essential fatty acids in health and chronic disease. *Am J Clin Nutr* 1999; 70(suppl): 560S–569S.
4. Cunnane S C, Zhen-Yu C, Yang J, *et al.* α-Linoleic acid in humans: direct functional role or dietary precursor? *Nutrition* 1991; 7: 437–439.
5. Cunnane S C. α-Linoleic acid in human nutrition and disease. *Nutrition* 1991; 7: 436.
6. De Lorgeril M, Renaud S, Mamelle N, *et al.* Mediterranean alpha-linoleic acid-rich diet in secondary prevention of coronary heart disease. *Lancet* 1994; 343: 1454–1459.
7. Harris W S. n-3 Fatty acids and serum lipoproteins: human studies. *Am J Clin Nutr* 1997; 65(suppl): 1645S–1654S.
8. Layne K S, Goh Y K, Jumpsen J A, *et al.* Normal subjects consuming physiological levels of 18:3(n-3) and 20:5(n-3) from flaxseed or fish oils have characteristic differences in plasma lipid and lipoprotein fatty acid levels. *J Nutr* 1996; 126: 2130–2140.
9. Allman M A, Pena N M, Pang D. Supplementation with flaxseed oil versus sunflower oil in healthy young men consuming a low fat diet: effects on platelet composition and function. *Eur J Clin Nutr* 1995; 49: 169–178.

10. Nestel P J, Pomeroy S E, Sasahara T, *et al.* Arterial compliance in obese subjects is improved with dietary plant n-3 fatty acid from flaxseed oil despite increased LDL oxidizability. *Arterioscler Thromb Vasc Biol* 1997; 17: 1163–1170.
11. Cunnane S C, Hamadeh M J, Liede A C, *et al.* Nutritional attributes of traditional flaxseed in healthy young adults. *Am J Clin Nutr* 1995; 61: 62–68.
12. Prassad K. Dietary flax seed in the prevention of hypercholesterolemic atherosclerosis. *Atherosclerosis* 1997; 132: 69–76.
13. Prassad K, Mantha S V, Muir A F, *et al.* Reduction of hypercholesterolemic atherosclerosis by CDC-flaxseed with very low alpha-linolenic acid. *Atherosclerosis* 1998; 136: 367–375.
14. Jenkins D J A, Kendall C W C, Vidgen E, *et al.* Health aspects of partially defatted flaxseed, including effects on serum lipids, oxidative measures, and *ex vivo* androgen and progestin activity: a controlled crossover trial. *Am J Clin Nutr* 1999; 69: 395–402.
15. Iso H, Rexrode K M, Stampfer M J, *et al.* Intake of fish and omega-3 fatty acids and risk of stroke in women. *JAMA* 2001; 285: 304–312.
16. Kelley D S, Branch L B, Love J E, *et al.* Dietary α-linoleic acid and immunocompetence in humans. *Am J Clin Nutr* 1991; 53: 40–46.
17. James M J, Gibson R A, Cleland L G. Dietary polyunsaturated fatty acids and inflammatory mediator production. *Am J Cin Nutr* 2000; 71(suppl): 343S–348S.
18. Clark W F, Parbtani A, Huff M W, *et al.* Flaxseed: a potential treatment for lupus nephritis. *Kidney Int* 1995; 48: 475–480.
19. Clark W F, Parbtani A. Proceedings from the National Kidney Foundation Annual Meeting: Symposium on essential fatty acid deficiencies and ω-3 unsaturated fat dietary supplementation in glomerulonephritis: basis and practice. *Am J Kidney Dis* 1994: 23: 644–647.
20. Clark W F, Muir A D, Westcott N D, *et al.* A novel treatment for lupus nephritis: lignan precursor derived from flax. *Lupus* 2000; 9: 429–436.
21. Nordstrom D C E, Honkanen V E A, Nasu Y, *et al.* Alpha-linolenic acid in the treatment of rheumatoid arthritis. A double-blind, placebo controlled and randomized study: flaxseed vs. safflower seed. *Rheumatol Int* 1995; 14: 231–234.
22. Caughey G E, Mantzioris E, Gibson R A, *et al.* The effect on human tumor necrosis factor α and interleukin 1β production of diets enriched in n-3 fatty acids from vegetable oil or fish oil. *Am J Clin Nutr* 1996; 63: 116–122.
23. Kremer J M. n-3 Fatty acid supplements in rheumatoid arthritis. *Am J Clin Nutr* 2000; 71(suppl): 349S–351S.
24. Ogborn M R, Nitschmann E, Weiler H, *et al.* Flaxseed ameliorates interstitial nephritis in rat polycystic kidney disease. *Kidney Int* 1999; 55: 417–423.
25. Nesbitt P D, Lam Y, Thompson L U. Human metabolism of mammalian lignan precursors in raw and processed flaxseed. *Am J Clin Nutr* 1999; 69: 549–555.
26. Thompson L U. Experimental studies on lignans and cancer. *Baillière's Clin Endocrinol Metab* 1998; 12: 691–705.
27. Brzezinski A, Debi A. Phytoestrogens: the 'natural' selective estrogen receptor modulators? *Eur J Obstet Gynecol Reprod Biol* 1999; 85: 47–51.
28. Phipps W R, Martini M C, Lampe J W, *et al.* Effect of flaxseed ingestion on the menstrual cycle. *J Clin Endocrinol Metab* 1993; 77: 1215–1219.

29. Albertazzi P, Pansini F, Bonaccorsi G, *et al.* The effect of dietary soy supplementation on hot flushes. *Obstet Gynecol* 1998; 91: 6–11.
30. Thompson L U, Rickard S E, Orcheson L J, *et al.* Flaxseed and its lignan and oil components reduce mammary tumour growth at a late stage of carcinogenesis. *Carcinogenesis* 1996; 17: 1373–1376.
31. Sung M K, Lautens M, Thompson L U. Mammalian lignans inhibit the growth of estrogen-independent human colon tumour cells. *Cancer Res* 1998; 18: 1405–1408.
32. Makrides M, Gibson R A. Long-chain polyunsaturated fatty acid requirements during pregnancy and lactation. *Am J Clin Nutr* 2000; 71(suppl): 307S–311S.
33. Uauy R, Hoffman D R. Essential fat requirements of preterm infants. *Am J Clin Nutr* 2000; 71(suppl): 245S–250S.
34. Mantzioris E, Cleland L G, Gibson R A, *et al.* Biochemical effects of a diet containing foods enriched with n-3 fatty acids. *Am J Clin Nutr* 2000; 72: 42–48.

# 8

# Melatonin

In the late 1990s the hormone melatonin became a very popular topic for discussion, with many articles being written about it both in the popular and scientific press. As well as books and papers, there are also Internet sites,[1] which are available to the health professional as well as to the general public. Despite the abundance of literature, however, it is often hard to differentiate between unproven myth and scientific fact, and pharmacists are in a good position to be able to answer questions about this supplement.

## Properties and structure

Melatonin (*N*-acetyl-5-methoxytryptamine) (Figure 8.1) is the primary hormone secreted by the pineal gland, which lies at the centre of the brain. The hormone was first identified in the late 1950s and it is biosynthesised from the amino acid tryptophan, via the intermediate serotonin. This biosynthesis and the subsequent release of melatonin is usually inhibited by exposure to light and stimulated by darkness, via a multisynaptic neural pathway, connecting the pineal gland to the retina.[2] However, the 24-hour cycle (or circadian rhythm) of melatonin secretion is endogenous in nature and is observed even when subjects are kept in constant darkness. Light seems to alter this rhythm rather than cause it.[3] Melatonin secretion usually starts as soon as darkness falls and usually peaks between 2 a.m. and 4 a.m.

The amount of melatonin produced varies with age. Babies secrete little melatonin, but from the age of about three months, melatonin concentrations begin to increase, being at a maximum between one and three years of age. Young adults secrete 5–25 μg of melatonin daily and this decreases markedly with advancing age.[4]

Melatonin is rapidly metabolised by the liver, with more than 85% being excreted as 6-sulfatoxymelatonin (6-SMT) in urine, which is used as a research tool to measure plasma melatonin.[5] Low doses of between 0.1 mg and 0.3 mg result in serum concentrations similar to the usual, physiological, night-time peak, but doses of between 1 and

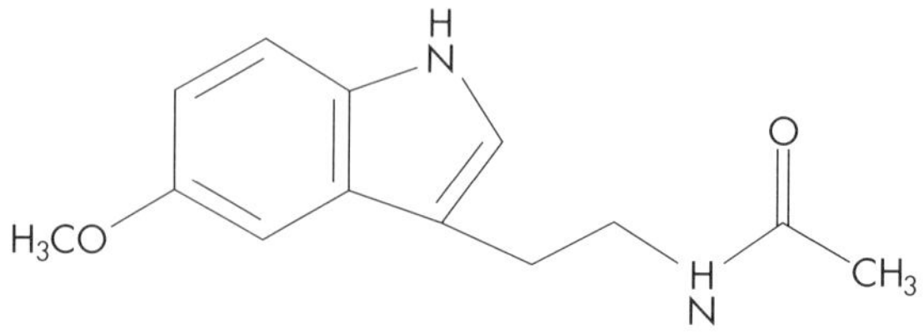

**Figure 8.1** Structure of melatonin.

5 mg (pharmacological doses) result in serum concentrations of up to 100 times higher than this concentration.[3] Oral doses of melatonin have a short half-life and are quickly cleared, and even very high nightly doses of 50 mg are cleared by the following morning. However, after two weeks of high daily dosing, lipid storage occurs.[4] Sustained-release preparations are available (in the USA) for a prolonged effect.[6]

Because it is a hormone, melatonin is usually referred to as a drug, but it is also a nutrient. The consumption of plant material containing high levels of melatonin could alter serum concentrations. Melatonin has been identified in bananas, tomatoes, cucumbers and beetroots, although massive amounts of these foods would have to be eaten to achieve pharmacological doses.[4,7] Doses of melatonin vary from 0.3 to 25 mg.[8]

## Legal requirements

Melatonin is a good example of a substance for which different countries have different regulations. In the UK, the Medicines Control Agency has restricted melatonin to prescription, available on a named patient basis only. There are no British licensed products, so it is unlawful to promote melatonin in this country. However, in the USA it may be sold as a food supplement or antioxidant, under the Dietary Supplement Health and Education Act of 1994, without approval from the Food and Drug Administration (FDA). British residents can legally bring melatonin purchased in the US back home for their personal use.[6]

## Uses of melatonin

Melatonin has been investigated for many different uses, based on its physiological roles. As it controls the circadian rhythms, it has been widely researched as an aid to prevent jet lag and for the alleviation of insomnia. Melatonin has also been found to be a powerful free-radical scavenger and as such its use as an antioxidant and in ageing has been studied. Leading on from this work, the role of melatonin in the immune system and in cancer has led to research in these areas too. Melatonin is also involved in seasonal breeding of animals and its effects on human reproduction have been studied. These research areas will be reviewed, with reference to some of the vast amount of literature found.

## Jet lag

Jet lag is a considerable problem in the modern world with the widespread use of air travel for both business and pleasure. When the internal body clock (or circadian rhythm) is not synchronised with the external 'local' time (light–dark cycle) jet lag is experienced. The symptoms, which vary between individuals, include tiredness, inability to sleep at the new bedtime, inability to concentrate and disturbed sleep for several days after a long flight, as well as headache and gastrointestinal problems. All of these, as well as the resulting sleep loss, can interfere with business meetings and pleasure activities. It may also cause considerable problems for training and performance in sports competitions and should be taken into account when planning journey times for sportsmen/women. Symptoms are more marked in older travellers and as more time zones are crossed, tending to be worse when travelling in an easterly direction.[9,10]

A chronobiotic is a class of drug that can alter the circadian rhythms, and melatonin falls in this class, as it is secreted during the night and affects the body clock.[10] Much research has been carried out using melatonin in the area of sleep disorders and jet lag. An early double-blind trial was carried out in 1986,[11] using 17 volunteers, between the ages of 29 and 68, who flew from London to San Francisco (eight time zones west). After 14 days, once the subjects had adapted to the local time, they were flown back to London. For three days before the return flight, a dose of 5 mg melatonin or placebo was taken at 6 p.m. local time and on return to Britain the dose was continued for a further four days, between 10 p.m. and midnight local time. On day 7 after arriving home, the subjects were asked to assess the jet lag they had experienced. It was found that none of the melatonin group had suffered appreciable jet lag, but six out of nine placebo subjects had. Although this study used a small sample of subjects and results were purely subjective, it showed the first promising results using melatonin for jet lag.

In another similar double-blind study,[12] 20 volunteers (aged 28–68) flew eastwards from Auckland, New Zealand to London, through 12 time zones, and returned after three weeks. Subjects took either placebo or 5 mg melatonin for the first journey and the other for the second journey, in a double-blind test. Less jet lag was experienced in the travellers taking melatonin than in the placebo group. The dose of 5 mg melatonin was well tolerated with few side-effects reported (a mild sedative effect in two subjects and a relaxed feeling in another). As in the former study the results were favourable, but more research was necessary to determine the optimum dose and dosing schedule. Also, the symptoms of jet lag were not standardised in either study and were subjective, making comparisons difficult. However, baseline symptoms, such as previous fatigue, stress due to travel preparations and the flight itself, or inability to sleep in a new environment or due to business or other activities, were not taken into account. Therefore it is hard to say which effects were due to the jet lag and improved specifically by melatonin.[9]

In a more recent study,[9] these problems were addressed. The sample size was large ($n$ = 257) and a scale was used to assess the severity of the jet lag experienced, including daytime symptoms, when travelling from New York to Oslo (six time zones eastwards). A randomised, double-blind procedure was used in which subjects received either placebo or 5 mg melatonin at bedtime, 0.5 mg melatonin at bedtime or 0.5 mg melatonin taken on a shifting schedule, starting at bedtime and taken one hour earlier each day. The results were somewhat surprising, with melatonin not showing significant improvement over placebo. However, the authors admit that the study had various limitations. Symptoms of sleep disturbance, which are associated with jet lag, were not examined, but rather daytime disturbance and times of sleep onset at night, and awakening in the morning. The reason for this was that results from the pilot study showed that these factors were less related to the overall assessment of disturbing jet lag. Also the subjects remained only four days in their destination before flying back and may not have fully adjusted to the local time. There may also have been a large placebo effect, as the subjects knew that they had three out of four chances of receiving melatonin, which would make the actual melatonin effect even smaller. The authors concluded that more work was needed to assess the use of melatonin in jet lag.

A recent Cochrane Review[13] assessed 9 trials comparing melatonin with placebo and one which compared it with the hypnotic zolpidem. In 9 out of 10 trials melatonin decreased jet lag resulting from crossing five or more time zones, when taken close to the desired bedtime at the destination (10pm to midnight). This excludes one trial which had a design fault,[9] and has been described above. A dose of 0.5mg was comparable to 5 mg in effect, but sleep was of faster onset and better quality with the 5 mg dose. A dose of 2 mg S/R melatonin was less effective than the short-lived higher peak concentration melatonin. The time of dosing was very important as if taken at the wrong time melatonin could cause a delay in adaptation to the local time. The safety profile was very high in these trials and the authors concluded that melatonin can safely be recommended to adults travelling across 5 or more time zones, particularly for those who have previously experienced jet lag.

## Sleep disorders

Sleep disturbances are very common, especially in the elderly. These can be primary, age-related disorders, or secondary to drugs, illness, anxiety or stress. Examples of these secondary causes include beta-blockers, pain and discomfort. Side-effects of drugs, such as increased urination, gastrointestinal effects and nausea can also interfere with sleep.[5] As melatonin is involved in the circadian rhythm and the sleep–wake cycle, it is logical that it might be used in the treatment of primary sleeping problems. It is important to eliminate secondary causes of sleep disorders as far as possible when recruiting volunteers for melatonin studies, to ensure that only the primary cause is being studied.

Six healthy, young men were used in a study to investigate the effect of melatonin given at night.[14] None of the subjects suffered from any sleep disorders or took any medication, and they refrained from alcohol and caffeine for 24 hours before each session. It was found that doses of 0.3 mg and 1 mg melatonin given at 8 p.m. or 9 p.m. produced acute hypnotic effects. These effects were assessed both subjectively and using polysomnographs (which use electroencephalographic electrodes). The authors suggested that a critical plasma melatonin level may be necessary for sleep induction. There was no residual hypnotic effect on the morning following melatonin administration, determined from mood and performance tests carried out by the volunteers. These results are promising for melatonin administration in insomniac patients.

In another study[15] involving 20 subjects that met the criteria for primary insomnia, plasma samples were taken every half-hour between 6.30 p.m. and 11 p.m., and radioimmunoassay was used to test for plasma melatonin. It was found that there were significantly lower concentrations of melatonin in the plasma of insomniacs than in the

20 controls matched for sex and age. This small study suggests that the lower plasma melatonin levels could have affected sleep in these subjects.

### The elderly

Melatonin has a half-life of only 40–50 minutes, with serum concentrations after oral dosing reaching peak levels after 20 minutes. Therefore, to ensure high serum levels throughout the night to ensure sleep maintenance as well as sleep initiation, either a very high dose would have to be given, or frequent, low-dose administration. A controlled-release tablet of 2 mg melatonin was formulated to overcome these problems and this was tested in 12 elderly insomniacs who were taking various medications for chronic illnesses (six had hypertension, five had ischaemic heart disease, four had spondyloarthrosis, three had Parkinson's disease and two had diabetes mellitus).[5] The patients, from a senior citizens home, were taking between one and six drugs (nitrates, calcium-channel blockers, diuretics, aspirin, beta-blockers and analgesics) and also used sleep medication.

Before starting the study, the subjects were woken every three hours during one night, to measure urinary 6-SMT. These results were compared with values from an earlier study by the authors involving elderly people without insomnia. In all subjects, the peak excretion of 6-SMT was between 3 a.m. and 6 a.m., rather than beginning at midnight as in young adults and elderly people without insomnia. This indicated that the sleep disorders might well be due to a shift in plasma melatonin secretion. Actigraphy was then used to assess sleep patterns for three nights. This method uses wrist movements to assess sleep patterns while the subject is in their own bed, which makes it a good tool for long-term studies in the elderly. To test the effect of melatonin supplements, a random, crossover design was used, in which the subjects were given 2 mg controlled-release melatonin, or placebo, 2 hours before bedtime, for three weeks. Actigraphy was used again for three nights at the end of the study.

Results showed an overall improvement in sleep quality in the subjects given melatonin, despite chronic disease states and concomitant medication. The authors explained these positive results as follows. First, as described above, it is necessary to establish melatonin deficiency in the subjects used. Also, the controlled-release formulation may have prevented desensitisation to large doses required for the same plasma concentration. A minimum of three weeks' treatment is also important, as it has been shown in animal studies that melatonin receptors can be reduced in the elderly and need to be resensitised by long-term exposure. A further reason given is that the internal clock in the elderly is sometimes not synchronised with the light–dark cycle and exogenous melatonin will correct this over a few weeks.

### *Visually impaired children*

Various studies of the effects of melatonin on visually impaired children have been reviewed.[8] In one such study, 2.5–10 mg melatonin given orally at bedtime improved sleep patterns with no side-effects in 70 children and also made the children more alert, more sociable and increased development. In another reported study, oral melatonin was used to successfully treat sleep–wake disturbances in six out of eight functionally blind children, who did not see the light–dark changes, which would usually stimulate melatonin secretion. The effect was maintained between 1 and 6 years.[8]

An interesting case has been reported[16] of a young woman who suffered excessive drowsiness, which became more severe after childbirth. At age 13 she had undergone partial resection of what was thought to be a pinealoma. On admission to hospital, at age 24, the woman spent most of the day sleeping. Urinary melatonin levels were found to be very low and unrelated to circadian rhythms. After eight weeks on 2 mg melatonin at night, the patient showed usual sleep patterns, with only a 20-minute nap during the day. It was interesting to note the increased severity of somnolence following pregnancy, which improved with melatonin therapy.

### *Neurological disorders*

There is a rare genetic disorder called Angelman's syndrome (AS), which is characterised by many symptoms including mental retardation and hyperactivity. Disturbed initiation and maintenance of sleep, which is difficult to treat using traditional sedatives in these patients, is also evident. This normally starts at a few months of age and may cause severe problems for the patient and carers. In a recent study the use of melatonin in AS was investigated.[17] Low-dose (0.3 mg) melatonin was given to 13 children, 30–60 minutes before their usual bedtime, for six nights. There was an improvement in sleep patterns, combined with a reduction of motor activity during the sleep period. This was accompanied by moderate increases in melatonin levels. Twelve out of

13 parents agreed to extend the study for a year. This study showed the possible benefits of small increases in melatonin levels in AS children.

In a similar, small study[18] to treat circadian rhythm sleep disorders in handicapped children, 3 mg melatonin was given at bedtime for between 4 and 12 months. The ten children involved in this open, prospective trial had suffered from sleep disorders for at least six months and had not responded to at least one hypnotic drug. Most of the children had epilepsy and visual impairment. The melatonin was well tolerated, causing no side-effects, and led to a dramatic response in eight out of ten of the children.

Another study involved ten children who were all being treated with a combination of antiepileptic drugs and who suffered from sleep–wake disturbances.[19] One hour before bedtime the children received 5 mg melatonin. If no response was seen after three to five days, the dose was increased to a maximum of 10 mg. Two children responded well to the 5 mg dose, and a further six responded well to the increased dose. As well as better sleep throughout the night, these children were also more alert and receptive during the day. In the two remaining children, when there was no response from 5 mg, the parents refused to increase the dose to 10 mg. Six of the children also showed a definite decrease in seizure frequency as a result of melatonin therapy. The authors suggested that this may have been an indirect result, since sleep disturbances activate seizures. Alternatively, melatonin may have had a direct action on brain tissue, resulting in suppressed epileptic activity.

The effects of melatonin have also been studied in 11 patients with intractable epilepsy.[20] These patients suffer from seizures, sleep disorders and lethargy following seizures, which can last a few days. Baseline melatonin levels for the test group were less than those of controls, but following a seizure these levels increased. The low starting melatonin level may reflect a disorder in neurological function and the authors suggested that the surge in melatonin following a seizure might be a protective mechanism to prevent further seizures. Melatonin supplements may be of use in such patients.

This research may also be of benefit in other neurological conditions in which sleep disturbances are present, but far more studies on larger groups of patients are required. However, it must be noted that some reviews have reported adverse effects in epileptic patients, and therefore caution must be exercised in such patients when using melatonin.[13]

### Ageing and antioxidant properties

In a remarkable experiment, the pineal glands were removed from young adult (3–4 month) and old (18 month), genetically pure, inbred mice and cross-transplanted.[21] Control mice were operated on in the same way, but the original pineal gland was replaced. Physical conditions, body weight and lifespan were then compared in the mice. A significant increase of ageing and death was seen in the mice transplanted with an 'old' pineal gland while in the old mice transplanted with a 'young' pineal gland, ageing and death were slowed. In both cases the difference in ageing was by six months, a quarter of the lifespan of that strain of mice. This experiment clearly demonstrates the importance of the pineal gland in ageing and death.

A study of 60 human subjects,[22] who were healthy and took no medication for one month prior to the start of the trial, was carried out to determine how melatonin production differed with age. Total daily melatonin production was found using a sensitive assay for the urinary metabolite 6-hydroxymelatonin. Urine samples were collected from 5 p.m. until 10 a.m., over three consecutive nights around midsummer. This was then repeated in midwinter. The results showed no statistical difference between summer and winter, but when the correlation was determined between age, sex, height and weight, melatonin production was found to decrease with age. The mechanisms for this may include calcification of the pineal gland or a decreased amount of β-adrenergic receptors, both of which have been found in aged rodents. It is therefore imperative that any trials for melatonin should use subjects matched for age. In much of the literature found for melatonin, this was not the case and could explain inconsistent results.

In addition to the decrease of melatonin with age, degenerative diseases increase with age. The increasing amount of evidence in both of these areas strongly indicates that there is a definite relationship between degenerative disease and decreased melatonin production. Accumulated oxidative stress, as a result of free radical reactions, is a major theory to explain ageing and age-related disease (as described in Chapter 4). When endogenous antioxidants are depleted or when free radicals increase, both of which can occur due to toxins, and in advancing age, then oxidative damage occurs. This leads to degeneration of cells and organs, resulting in loss of function and disease. Both endogenous antioxidants, such as glutathione, and exogenous supplements, like vitamin C and vitamin E, are important to prevent oxidative damage.[23]

Since melatonin had been reported to have anti-ageing properties and protective properties against cell damage, it was speculated that melatonin may exhibit antioxidant properties, since oxidation was common to both anti-ageing and cell degeneration. In 1993 melatonin was indeed found to act as a scavenger of the hydroxyl radical.[24] This is one of the principal reactive free radicals in living organisms and it causes oxygen toxicity by generating other reactive species, eventually causing cell degeneration and death. It was also found that melatonin did not show any pro-oxidant effects, unlike other antioxidants, such as vitamin C, which are either pro-oxidant or antioxidant depending on the physiological conditions. The research indicated that at high concentrations, melatonin was a potent antioxidant, with high lipophilicity, enabling it to enter all cellular compartments, with no toxicity. However, the experiments using melatonin were carried out *in vitro* and at concentrations far exceeding those found under normal conditions, so that conclusions about whether this is an important role at physiological levels cannot be made.

Much work has been published investigating the role of melatonin in scavenging many other reactive species, besides the hydroxyl radical, as well as its ability to stabilise lipid membranes, enabling them to resist oxidative damage. This action of melatonin is independent of any receptor binding and may be partly due to the stimulation of intracellular antioxidants, such as glutathione and inhibition of oxidising enzymes, such as nitric oxide synthase. Reiter provides a detailed review of melatonin and its antioxidant properties.[25]

As already stated, the pharmacological doses used to achieve antioxidation are far higher than the endogenous, physiological concentrations present in the body. Furthermore, most studies to date have used animal models in the research, rather than human studies.[3,25] The application to humans, therefore, must be considered with caution. It is too early to promote the use of melatonin as an anti-ageing supplement, but its low toxicity and high lipophilicity makes it a good choice for further research.

## Cancer and enhanced immunity

As well as showing antioxidant properties, which may have an effect on the spread of cancer cells, melatonin has shown direct inhibition of various cancer cells both *in vitro* and *in vivo*.[2] There is conflicting evidence for the role of melatonin in cancer therapy, but the majority of studies show positive results, and a low level of endogenous melatonin has been shown in women with breast cancer and in men with prostatic cancer.[3] Melatonin has been beneficial in many different cancers, including breast cancer, non-small cell lung cancer, metastatic renal cell carcinoma, hepatocellular carcinoma and brain metastases due to solid tumours. In most of these studies melatonin was given at a large dose of between 10 mg and 50 mg daily.

A group of 80 patients, with advanced solid tumours who refused chemotherapy or who did not respond to previous chemotherapy were entered into a study.[26] Low-dose interleukin 2 (IL-2) anti-tumour immunotherapy has been used to treat cancers, since cells involved in cancer cell destruction are controlled by this cytokine. In spite of this, it has been found that few cancers respond well to IL-2 alone. In this study melatonin was added to the treatment regimen to see if its effect enhanced the IL-2 response. The patients randomly received either IL-2 alone for four weeks, or were supplemented with 40 mg melatonin daily at 8 p.m. for six days a week, starting one week before the IL-2 treatment period. After a rest period of three weeks, a second treatment month was given and thereafter the patients received a maintenance treatment for one week each month. The addition of melatonin increased the anti-tumour activity of low-dose IL-2, resulting in an accelerated tumour regression rate, increased progression-free survival and longer overall survival in these patients, as defined by WHO criteria. The occurrence of side-effects was low in both groups, with no significant difference between the two. A similar trial was carried out involving 14 patients with haematologic malignancies, for whom no other treatment was available.[27] Again low-dose IL-2 in combination with melatonin was well tolerated and effective and prolonged survival time in previously untreatable patients.

There has been much *in vitro* work carried out on breast cancer cells. Although some groups have not found an inhibitory effect with melatonin, most have.[28] One research group has shown that there may be benefits to giving melatonin together with retinoic acid.[30] Retinoids have been shown to inhibit breast cancer cell lines *in vitro* but clinical use is limited by their toxicity. In animal models the combination of retinoic acid and melatonin reduced the growth of mammary tumours.

In a small-scale human study,[31] melatonin was given to 14 women with metastatic breast cancer who did not respond to tamoxifen therapy or who progressed after initial stabilisation. Melatonin was started seven days before the tamoxifen treatment and was given at a dose of 20 mg each evening. The addition of melatonin increased the response to tamoxifen resulting in tumour regression. Again there was no toxicity reported.

In patients with solid neoplasms, brain metastases present a very serious condition. Although chemotherapy and radiation therapy have been tried, there is no clear prolongation of survival time, which is often less than six months in these patients. A study was performed on 50 such patients.[32] They were treated by supportive measures (steroids and anticonvulsants) alone or with the addition of 20 mg melatonin daily. Survival at one year was significantly higher in the patients receiving melatonin. Other benefits of the melatonin treatment included a clear improvement in the quality of life and a reduced frequency of steroid complications, as compared with the group receiving supportive care alone. This study justifies further work in this area, and large clinical trials to evaluate the use of melatonin in different types of cancer as clearly needed.

These small investigations show preliminary, positive results for a role of melatonin in cancer therapy, but large clinical trials are required to provide conclusive evidence. It is possible that melatonin exerts its anti-cancer properties through the immune system. It has been shown that melatonin enhances immune responses.[3,33] This is even more pronounced in immunocompromised states, including those resulting from stress, corticosteroid therapy or viral disease. Melatonin also seems to protect the cells against damage from cytotoxic agents and this may be due to antioxidant effects at the DNA level, due to its high intranuclear concentration.[25] However, care is needed before treatment is considered as it can worsen conditions such as autoimmune diseases, immune system cancers or severe allergies.[34]

## Reproduction

In jet lag studies it was noticed that the symptoms varied with the menstrual cycle. Also, air stewardesses often find that their cycles are irregular,[10] suggesting that disturbances of melatonin levels may also influence the menstrual cycle. Under normal circumstances melatonin levels do not change throughout the menstrual cycle, but few studies have been carried out to determine the effect of melatonin on the human reproductive system. In one interesting experiment using young women, a large dose of 300 mg melatonin daily for four months suppressed the midcycle surge in luteinizing hormone (LH) and partially inhibited ovulation. This effect was increased by the addition of a progestin minipill. Side-effects with this contraceptive use of melatonin included abnormal bleeding and headaches, but interestingly, no effect on sleep was reported.[3,35]

Most studies on reproduction and melatonin have been carried out in animals, as many animals have a seasonal reproduction cycle, which may be affected by melatonin levels. The role of melatonin in non-seasonal breeders, such as humans, has not been defined but should be considered when starting melatonin therapy.[2] It has been suggested that the onset of puberty is related to the decrease of melatonin as children grow, since children who show early puberty have low levels of melatonin and some children showing very early puberty have been found to have low levels of melatonin for their age.[3]

### Other uses

There are reports of melatonin use in other situations. Many of these are based on animal studies and have insufficient evidence in humans. Examples include lowering cholesterol, treating coronary heart disease and alleviating cluster headaches.[2]

Melatonin has also been implicated in seasonal affective disorder (SAD), which is a syndrome affecting people in the winter and usually involving depression, fatigue, social withdrawal, oversleeping, overeating and weight gain. Bright light treatment and/or the onset of spring usually alleviate these symptoms.[36]

A novel use of melatonin has also been described,[37] in which melatonin was used in the reversal of morphine dependence in mice.

## Drug interactions

It is not advisable for melatonin to be taken with tranquillisers or antidepressants.[6] Benzodiazepines are reported to decrease night-time melatonin levels and increase daytime levels. This could explain the residual effect of benzodiazepines felt the following morning and could also be related to the rebound insomnia following withdrawal of treatment.[14] Interactions between melatonin and vitamin K antagonists such as warfarin may be life-threatening and until more research is carried out this combination should be avoided.[13]

Synthesis and release of melatonin are influenced by beta$_1$-adrenoceptors and alpha$_1$-adrenoceptors. This could explain the fact that beta-blockers are known to cause sleep disturbances, but particular stereochemical forms are necessary to test this hypothesis. In a study of 15 healthy males, it was found that 40 mg (*S*)-propranolol and 50 mg (*S*)-atenolol reduced nocturnal melatonin levels by specific inhibition of adrenergic beta$_1$-receptors when the pure enantiomers were given. The

(*R*)- forms and (*RS*)-carvedilol and (*RS*)-verapamil did not show the same results.[38] This indicated that a blockage of adrenoceptors was probably responsible, rather than the reduction of blood pressure.

In another study,[39] a significant reduction of melatonin levels was reported only after using metoprolol and not with atenolol or propranolol (although all resulted in lower melatonin levels). In this study subjects were not matched for age, sex and severity of hypertension, so the results are equivocal. There may be a place for the use of melatonin to avoid sleep disturbances in beta-blocker users, but further clinical trials are necessary.

Other commonly used drugs have also caused a decrease in nocturnal melatonin secretion. Examples include fluoxetine,[40] and the non-steroidal anti-inflammatory drugs indometacin and ibuprofen.[41]

Many melatonin preparations available may be contaminated by tryptophan-related substances, and should therefore be avoided in patients taking monoamine oxidase inhibitors (MAOIs).[34]

Two small studies found that oral ethanol, producing mild intoxication, inhibits melatonin levels. This may be part of the reason that ethanol causes sleep disturbances, including increased readiness to fall asleep but poorer sleep quality.[42,43] The disturbance in endogenous rhythms after mild or moderate intoxication may be the cause of altered mental alertness and increased fatigue on the morning following alcohol ingestion.

## Side-effects and contraindications

Melatonin is generally considered to be very safe. It has been argued that even in very high doses (300 mg/day) melatonin is safer than many over-the-counter remedies presently on sale. With correct use and necessary caution melatonin has a very high safety record.[7]

A study was carried out to assess the sleep-related aspects and side-effects of melatonin in 30 healthy, male volunteers who received 10 mg melatonin daily for 28 days, one hour before bedtime, as well as the effects on several urinary and biochemical parameters.[29] These included complete blood count, urine analysis, sodium, potassium and calcium levels, albumin, blood glucose, cholesterol values, urea, creatinine, thyroxine levels, uric acid, bilirubin, alkaline phosphate, glutamic-pyruvate transaminase (GPT), glutamic-oxalacetic transaminase (GOT), gamma-glutamic transaminase (GGT) and alkaline phosphatase levels. The results were compared with those from ten controls who received placebo. A feeling of sleepiness ($n$ = 17) and headache ($n$ = 14) were the two most pronounced side-effects in the group of 30 taking melatonin. However, these two effects were also reported in the placebo group and there was no statistical significant difference between the two groups. No other toxicological effects were noted for any of the parameters assessed for the melatonin group. Although this study indicated that melatonin is safe at the dose used for one month, long-term data on safety are not yet available.

In the USA, elderly insomniacs use melatonin freely. This leads to cause for concern as insomnia is often part of a depressive disorder, which melatonin could worsen.[4]

Effects on mental performance with doses of 5 mg have been reported, but if the subject is allowed to sleep after melatonin ingestion then no residual effects are noticed on waking.[10] In ten years of jet lag studies, Arendt, a leading researcher of jet lag, has found that daytime sleepiness occurs in about 8% of subjects given a 5-mg dose.[4] In one study of 572 subjects, one traveller reported symptoms of difficulty breathing and swallowing within 20 minutes of taking 0.5 mg melatonin, which lasted for 45 minutes. After the study, the subject took another dose and similar, but milder symptoms occurred.[9]

There are conflicting reports of the side-effects of using melatonin for insomnia. Some studies suggest that melatonin is very safe even in high doses,[4] and others claim that in 10% of people using melatonin at high dose, insomnia and nightmares have resulted.[34] Although the dose required to induce sleep is between 0.1 and 0.3 mg, doses of 2–3 mg are available.

The effect of melatonin on driving performance has been studied, with the overall result being that melatonin did not adversely affect driving ability. However, caution should be exercised when driving after taking melatonin, due to the increased sleepiness which may occur.[44]

In a study in the elderly, pruritis was noted in one out of 12 participants taking 2 mg melatonin each night for three weeks.[5]

An unusual side-effect has been reported recently.[45] A man suffering with amyotrophic lateral sclerosis (ALS), a degenerative motor neuron disease involving a group of chronic neurological disorders affecting the spinal cord and lower brainstem, developed painful gynaecomastia. The patient had been taking melatonin 1 mg/day increasing to 2 mg/day in the last 18 months, as well as riluzole, citalopram and vitamin E. On stopping the melatonin, symptoms spontaneously resolved. This is an interesting case and demonstrates that the absence of side-effects in the healthy population does not necessarily mean that melatonin is safe for everyone.

It is also worth noting that since animal studies have shown the potential for cardiovascular effects, those self-medicating with melatonin should be aware of the possibility of such effects in humans, which are of particular importance to heart patients.[46]

## Conclusions

In general, melatonin can be thought of as a beneficial and safe supplement, but caution must always be employed before starting therapy. The minimum dose should be used in each case and the following groups of patients should avoid its use:

- Women wishing to conceive or those breastfeeding babies. Maternal melatonin crosses the placenta and therefore should be avoided in women wishing to conceive and in pregnancy.[43] There are melatonin receptors in the fetus from an early stage of development and high placental melatonin concentrations may lead to fetal abnormalities.
- People with allergies or autoimmune disease.
- Children, who have naturally high melatonin levels.
- Patients with severe mental illness.
- Patients taking MAOIs.
- Patients taking warfarin.

If the present interest in melatonin continues then the many unanswered questions as to its place as either a nutraceutical or indeed as a licensed medicine may begin to be answered. Melatonin certainly seems to be an interesting substance, which, with cautious use, has many benefits.

## References

1. The complete reference centre and information source for melatonin. http://www.melatonin.com (accessed 1 September 2001).
2. Birdsall T C. The biological effects and clinical uses of the pineal hormone melatonin. *Altern Med Rev* 1996; 1: 94–101.
3 Brzezinski A. Melatonin in humans. *N Engl J Med* 1997; 336: 186–195.
4. Lamberg L. Melatonin potentially useful but safety, efficacy remain uncertain. *JAMA* 1996; 276: 1011–1014.
5. Garfinkle D, Laudon M, Nof D, *et al.* Improvement of sleep quality in elderly people by controlled-release melatonin. *Lancet* 1995; 346: 541–544.
6. Gladwin C. Time capsule. *Chemist Druggist* 1997; 2 August: v–vii.
7. Moss J. Melatonin revisited – what is it? *Altern Ther Clin Pract* 1996; 3: 11–14.

8. Gordon N. The therapeutics of melatonin: a paediatric perspective. *Brain Dev* 2000; 22: 213–217.
9. Spitzer R L, Terman M, Williams J B W, *et al.* Jet lag: clinical features, validation of a new syndrome-specific scale, and lack of response to melatonin in a randomised, double-blind trial. *Am J Psychiatry* 1999; 156: 1392–1396.
10. Waterhouse J, Reilly T, Atkinson G. Jet lag. *Lancet* 1997; 350: 1611–1615.
11. Arendt J, Aldhous M, Marks V. Alleviation of jet lag by melatonin: preliminary results of controlled double blind trial. *BMJ* 1986; 292: 1170.
12. Petrie K, Conaglen J V, Thompson L, *et al.* Effect of melatonin on jet lag after long haul flights. *BMJ* 1989; 298: 705–707.
13. Herxheimer A, Petrie K J. Melatonin for the prevention and treatment of jet lag (Cochrane Review). In: The Cochrane Library, Issue 3. Oxford: Update Software, 2001.
14. Zhdanova I V, Wurtman R J, Lynch H J, *et al.* Sleep inducing effects of low doses of melatonin ingested in the evening. *Clin Pharmacol Ther* 1995; 57: 552–558.
15. Attenburrow M E J, Dowling B A, Sharpley A L, *et al.* Case-control study of evening melatonin concentration in primary insomnia. *BMJ* 1996; 312: 1263–1264.
16. Lehmann E D, Cockerell O C, Rudge P. Somnolence associated with melatonin deficiency after pinealectomy. *Lancet* 1996; 347: 323.
17. Zhdanova I V, Wurtman R J, Wagstaff J. Effects of a low dose of melatonin on sleep in children with Angelman Syndrome. *J Pediatr Endocrinol Metab* 1999; 12: 57–67.
18. Jan M M. Melatonin for the treatment of handicapped children with severe disorders. *Pediatr Neurol* 2000; 23: 229–232.
19. Fauteck J D, Schmidt H, Lerchl A, *et al.* Melatonin in epilepsy: first results of replacement therapy and first clinical results. *Biol Signals Recept* 1999; 8: 105–110.
20. Bazil C W, Short D, Crispin D, *et al.* Patients with intractable epilepsy have low melatonin, which increases following seizures. *Neurology* 2000; 55: 1746–1748.
21. Lesnikov V A, Pierpaoli W. Pineal cross-transplantation (old to young and vice versa) as evidence for an endogenous 'aging clock'. *Ann NY Acad Sci* 1994; 719: 456–460.
22. Sack R L, Lewy A J, Erb D L, *et al.* Human melatonin production decreases with age. *J Pineal Res* 1986; 3: 379–388.
23. German J B, Dillard C J. Phytochemicals and targets of chronic disease. In: Bidlack W R, Omaye S T, Meskin M S, *et al.*, eds. *Phytochemicals. A New Paradigm.* Pennsylvania: Technomic Publishing, 1998: 13–32.
24. Tan D X, Chen L D, Poeggeler B, *et al.* Melatonin: a potent, endogenous hydroxyl radical scavenger. *Endocrinol J* 1993; 1: 57–60.
25. Reiter R J. Cytoprotective properties of melatonin: presumed association with oxidative damage and ageing. *Nutrition* 1998; 14: 691–696.
26. Lissoni P, Barni S, Tancini G, *et al.* A randomised study with subcutaneous low-dose interleukin 2 alone vs. interleukin 2 plus the pineal neurohormone melatonin in advanced solid neoplasms other than renal cancer and melanoma. *Br J Cancer* 1994; 69: 196–199.
27. Lissoni P, Bolis S, Brivio F, *et al.* A phase II study of neuroimmunotherapy with

subcutaneous low-dose IL-2 plus the pineal hormone melatonin in untreatable advanced hematologic malignancies. *Anticancer Res* 2000; 20: 2103–2106.
28. Ram P T, Yuan L, Dai J, *et al.* Differential responsiveness of MCF-7 human breast cancer cell line stocks to the pineal hormone, melatonin. *J Pineal Res* 2000; 28: 210–218.
29. Seabra M L V, Bignotto M, Pinto L R Jr, *et al.* Randomized, double-blind clinical trial, controlled with placebo, of the toxicology of chronic melatonin treatment. *J Pineal Res* 2000; 29: 193–200.
30. Hill S M, Teplitzky S, Ram P T, *et al.* Melatonin synergizes with retinoic acid in the prevention and regression of breast cancer. *Adv Exp Med Biol* 1999; 460: 345–362.
31. Lissoni P, Barni S, Meregalli S, *et al.* Modulation of cancer endocrine therapy by melatonin: a phase II study of tamoxifen plus melatonin in metastatic breast cancer patients progressing under tamoxifen alone. *Br J Cancer* 1995; 71: 854–856.
32. Lissoni P, Barni S, Ardizzoia A, *et al.* A randomised study with the pineal hormone melatonin versus supportive care alone in patients with brain metastases due to solid neoplasms. *Cancer* 1994; 73: 699–701.
33. Reiter R J, Maestroni G J M. Melatonin in relation to the antioxidative defense and immune systems: possible implications for cell and organ transplantation. *J Mol Med* 1999; 77: 36–39.
34. Priorities (1995). Herbert V, Kava R. The miracle of melatonin? http://www.hcrc.org/contrib/acsh/articles/melaton.html (accessed 17 February 2000).
35. Arendt J. Melatonin – claims made in the popular media are mostly nonsense. *BMJ* 1996; 312: 1242–1243.
36. Putilov A A, Russkikh G S, Danilenko K V. Phase of melatonin rhythm in winter depression. *Adv Exp Med Biol* 1999; 460: 441–458.
37. Raghavendra V, Shrinivas K, Kulkarni K. Reversal of morphine tolerance and dependence by melatonin: possible role of central and peripheral benzodiazepine receptors. *Brain Res* 1999; 834: 178–181.
38. Stoschitzky K, Sakotnik A, Lercher P, *et al.* Influence of beta blockers on melatonin release. *Eur J Clin Pharmacol* 1999; 55: 111–115.
39. Brismar K, Hylander B, Eliasson K, *et al.* Melatonin secretion related to side effects of beta blockers from the central nervous system. *Acta Med Scand* 1988; 223: 525–530.
40. Childs P A, Rodin I, Martin N J, *et al.* Effect of fluoxetine on melatonin in patients with seasonal affective disorder and matched controls. *Br J Psychiatry* 1995; 166: 196–198.
41. Surrall K, Smith J A, Bird H, *et al.* Effect of indometacin on human plasma melatonin. *J Pharm Pharmacol* 1987; 39: 840–843.
42. Rojdmark S, Wikner J, Adner N, *et al.* Inhibition of melatonin secretion by ethanol in man. *Metabolism* 1993; 42: 1047–1051.
43. Ekman A C, Leppaluoto J, Huttunen P, *et al.* Ethanol inhibits melatonin secretion in healthy volunteers in a dose-dependent randomised double blind cross-over study. *J Clin Endocr Metab* 1993; 77: 780–783.
44. Wetterberg L. Melatonin and clinical application. *Reprod Nutr Dev* 1999; 39: 367–382.

45. De Bleecker J L, Lamont B H, Verstraete A G, *et al.* Melatonin and painful gynecomastia. *Neurology* 1999; 53: 435–436.
46. Krause D N, Geary G G, Doolen S, *et al.* Melatonin and cardiovascular function. *Adv Exp Med Biol* 1999; 460: 299–310.

# 9

# Ornithine alpha ketoglutarate

Ornithine alpha ketoglutarate (OKG) is a supplement widely promoted for athletes, bodybuilders and sportsmen/women. Although the amino acids that comprise OKG are present in protein foods such as meat, poultry and fish, the OKG compound is found only in supplements. Medical evidence for this use is sparse and no matches were found on a Medline search for 'ornithine alpha ketoglutarate and athletes' and 'ornithine alpha ketoglutarate and sports'. A non-scientific Internet search led to many claims for the use of OKG for improving performance of athletes, but with no evidence. One such site stated 'there is little or no scientific evidence supporting positive effects on muscle growth, body fat reduction, or strength enhancement in strength-trained athletes'.[1]

Most studies that have been carried out address the medical and clinical uses of OKG, which is involved in protein metabolism. Supplementation by this means has also been called artificial or pharmacological nutrition.[2] In addition to its functions as a pharmacological nutrient, OKG also has a role in the secretion of some hormones and in the immune system.[3] OKG has been included here, as it is an interesting nutraceutical that could be used more in a hospital setting than by self-selection from pharmacies or health-food shops. In addition to a general description of OKG and its role in protein metabolism, evidence from animal and human studies will be reviewed, and some of the important uses in which OKG is being applied in medical practice will be discussed.

## Properties and structure

OKG is a salt formed from one molecule of alpha ketoglutarate (αKG) and two molecules of ornithine (Figure 9.1). It is a precursor of many metabolites including the amino acids glutamine, arginine and proline as well as the polyamines that are involved in cell propagation and tissue repair.[2,4]

In malnutrition states, the physiological glutamine pool is depleted. It cannot be replaced by glutamine, as this amino acid is poorly stable

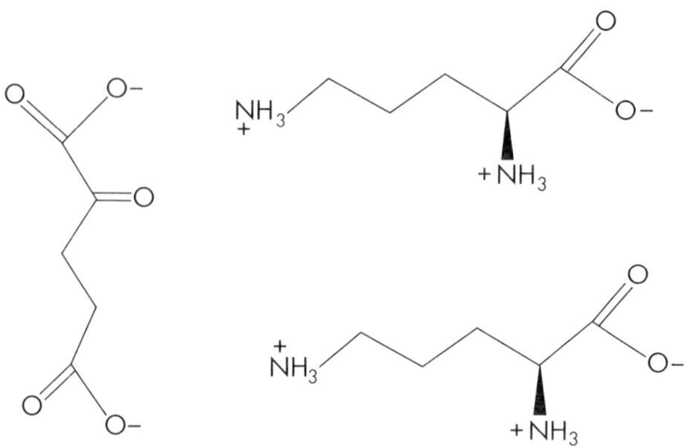


**Figure 9.1** Ornithine alpha ketoglutarate (OKG) is formed from two molecules of ornithine and one molecule of alpha ketoglutarate.[5]

in solution and in heat sterilisation, and is therefore unsuitable for clinical practice. Glutamate peptides are an expensive research tool and glutamate also gained bad publicity in the 'Chinese restaurant syndrome' when it was found to induce neurotoxicity in certain subjects who consumed Chinese food rich in glutamate. Therefore αKG is used as a precursor for glutamine. αKG has important functions in amino acid and protein metabolism and regulation.[5]

OKG was first used in the 1960s, when elevated ammonia levels were thought to be the major cause of coma. It was thought that OKG could be administered to such coma patients and in theory, the αKG would trap the ammonia and form glutamate. This would then enter the ureagenesis pathway, activated by ornithine. Although clinical results were disappointing, it was noticed that there was an increase in nutritional status (nitrogen balance and plasma amino acids) in the treated patients. This was the start of pharmacological nutrition using OKG, which was further developed in the mid-1980s and has since been used in many other clinical states with promising results.[3]

OKG is available in two forms, both supplied by Laboratoires J. Logeais, France. The freeze-dried powder ('Ornicetil') is used for parenteral administration and the hydrated form ('Cetornan') is used for oral and enteral use.

### Metabolic pathways

Ornithine is an amino acid involved in the urea cycle, where it is metabolised to citrulline and then to arginine, which in turn is regenerated to ornithine with the release of urea (Figure 9.2). It can also be metabolised to the polyamines (putrescine, spermine and spermidine) which are important in the processes of cell propagation and tissue repair.[4] Ornithine can be reversibly metabolised to glutamate. When it

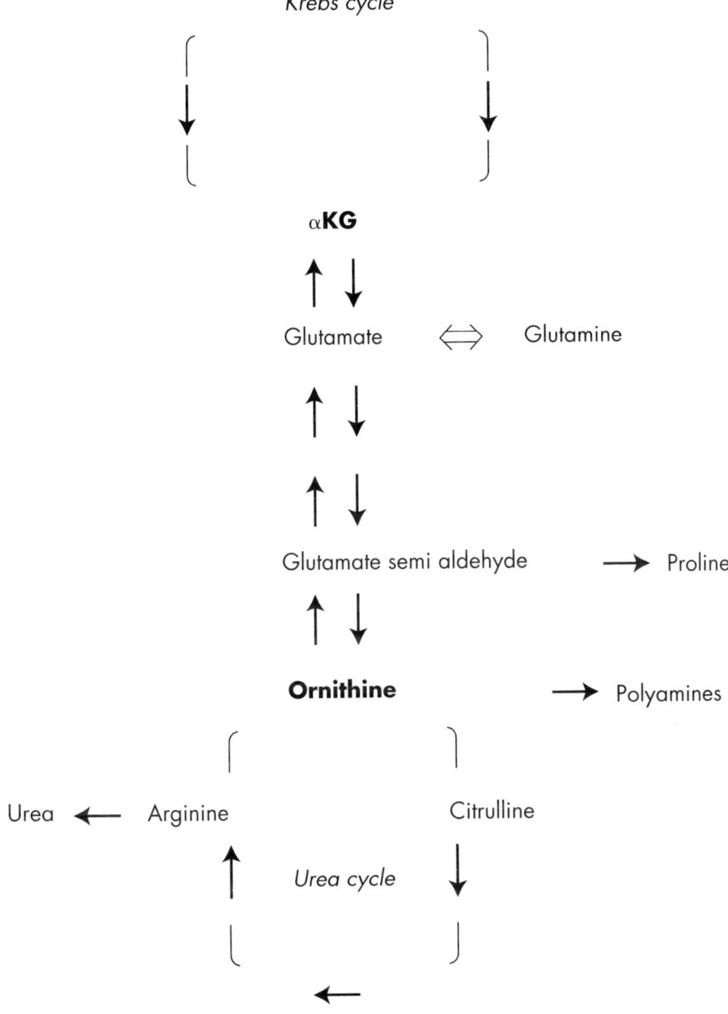


**Figure 9.2** The metabolic pathways of ornithine and alpha ketoglutarate.[2,3]

is converted to glutamate, the amino group is in the α position, which is the position favoured in the synthesis of most other amino acids. When glutamine synthase reacts with glutamate, glutamine is formed. Most of these reactions occur in muscle but some take place in liver and lung tissue.[6]

A small experiment was carried out to determine whether ornithine and αKG act independently or as part of the same pathways.[7] The results indicated that amino acid modification occurs only when OKG is given as one entity; when ornithine was given as the hydrochloride and αKG as the calcium salt, the same effects were not shown.

In another study to investigate which part of the OKG structure was the active moiety, an experiment was carried out in which rats were fed ornithine, αKG or OKG.[8] Forty-eight rats were divided into two groups, control and trauma. Each group was further subdivided into different isonitrogenous diets: basal, ornithine, αKG and OKG. The trauma group received a uniform closed fracture to the femur. All rats were then starved for two days and given only water to simulate conditions in trauma intensive care units. On day 3, each group began feeding on their specified diet and after four days the rats were analysed. Results were obtained for growth hormone and insulin secretion, nitrogen retention, free amino acids, proteolysis and protein synthesis, muscle glutamine concentration and muscle total amino acids. Overall, the authors concluded that there was a case for supplementation with OKG after severe injury rather than with its components ornithine and αKG.

## Mechanism of action

As already discussed, OKG exerts its actions through various pathways and metabolites:

- Glutamate is involved in nitrogen balance, important in malnutritional states and any situation where nitrogen balance is altered.
- Glutamine is an intermediary in protein metabolism and is used as an energy substrate and as a precursor of polyamines, which are involved in protein synthesis.
- Proline is another intermediary, involved in protein synthesis as well as in tissue repair and wound healing. Proline also affects hepatocyte DNA.
- Arginine is a semi-essential amino acid, being required only in young (growing) animals. In trauma states, when increased tissue synthesis is required, it becomes necessary again. Arginine also affects the secretion of insulin, glucagon and growth hormone, and OKG has been shown to affect these hormones, depending on the nutritional status of the subject.[3,5]

## Uses of OKG

OKG has been used in many experimental procedures, using both animal and human models. There are many disease states in which promising results have been found[3,9] and an overview is given below.

### Burn injury

Burn injury leads to a hormonal response resulting in weight decrease and body wasting as well as changes in amino acids in plasma and urine.[10,11] These changes correspond to the catabolism and anabolism (breakdown and synthesis) of proteins, resulting in a net negative nitrogen balance. In the first few hours after extensive burn injury, there is an increase in plasma ammonia and amino acids, as the wound proteins are broken down to provide substrate for energy production. Over time these return to normal, as part of the healing process. Reviews can be found in the literature assessing the role played by OKG in burn injury.[3,10]

In one study of 14 severely burned patients (burn surface area, BSA, was 16–31%), the test group received 10 g OKG each day, from day 2 to day 13 post injury, at which time most patients were discharged. These patients showed improved nitrogen balance over the control group.[12] In a similar study, 14 severely burned patients (BSA 21–60%) were studied, from day 4 to day 28 post injury.[11] The test group received 10 g OKG twice daily, by addition to the continuous feed. From plasma and urine amino acid measurements, the authors concluded that OKG limited the breakdown of protein via insulin and human growth hormone, rather than via its utilisation as energy source in the Krebs cycle.

To determine whether the metabolic changes observed resulted in improved clinical states, a two-year retrospective study was carried out involving 136 patients.[5] All patients were admitted within 48 hours of injury, received enteral nutrition, had similar BSA (>20%) and survived at least five days. In the patients receiving OKG supplementation, there was a mean reduction in hospital stay of 16 days, but this was statistically not significant, as there was wide variation between patients. There was, however, a trend towards a significant reduction in mortality in the OKG group.

In another experiment,[13] 60 patients who had severe burns (BSA 20–60%), were randomly divided between two groups. The test group received 20 g OKG, as two doses of 10 g daily, from day 1 to day 21, and the patients in the placebo group received an isocaloric placebo. Where possible the doses were oral, but otherwise they were via a nasogastric tube. Although at the beginning of the study patients in both groups showed similar clinical data and levels of injury, the patients in the OKG group showed a nitrogen-sparing effect from day 4. Moreover, weight loss was significantly lower in the treated group, and healing was quicker and of better quality. This indicated that the metabolic changes did influence the clinical outcome of such patients.

Burn patients have also been used to determine the optimum mode of administration (bolus or continuous) for OKG supplementary therapy, in two similar experiments.[4,14] Forty-two intensive care unit patients with BSA 20–50% were included in the first study. They were fed enterally and an OKG supplement or an isonitrogenous soy protein mixture as control was also given. To determine the dose–response for OKG, the patients received either 10 g daily as a bolus dose or 10 g, 20 g or 30 g as a continuous infusion, over 21 hours. This dose–response study could only be performed for the continuous feed patients, as bolus doses of more than 10 g resulted in diarrhoea. The OKG was rapidly and efficiently metabolised to glutamine, arginine and proline, determined from the analysis of blood samples. Glutamine and arginine production was influenced by the mode of administration, which was less in the bolus patients than in those given OKG by infusion. However proline production was not influenced by the mode of administration, and was dose-dependent. The authors suggested that a continuous infusion affected the equilibrium. Both ornithine and αKG can be metabolised through various pathways, and when administered together certain pathways are preferred through the saturation of others, and glutamine, arginine and polyamines are synthesised. However, when administered as a continuous infusion, smaller amounts of each moiety are available, shifting the equilibrium. When given as a continuous infusion it seems likely that the ornithine forms proline and the αKG forms glutamine, but when a bolus is given the excess ornithine available regenerates arginine and glutamine.

Forty-eight intensive-care burn patients were included in the second study[4] to compare the mode of administration and optimum dose for OKG supplementation. They were randomly divided into groups and given 10 g OKG daily, 10 g twice daily or 10 g three times daily as a bolus dose or the same doses by continuous infusion for 21 days after the burn injury. Again, controls using a soy protein mixture were also carried out. No difference was found between the body weight, tolerance (vomiting or diarrhoea), or number and length of septic episodes for any given dose or mode of administration. Bolus administration resulted in different metabolites being favoured as explained above, and an increase in glutamine concentration throughout the study. A shorter duration of enteral nutrition was necessary and length of hospital stay was reduced in the bolus patients, compared with continuous infusion. No conclusion was reached as to the optimum dose and further work is required in this area.

### Post surgery

OKG affects the low molecular weight polyamines (putrescine, spermidine and spermine) that are involved in cellular proliferation, cell growth and protein synthesis.[15] In trauma, cell breakdown and death are followed by the regeneration of tissues. This proteolysis, lipolysis and gluconeogenesis leads to an increase of extracellular polyamines and increased polyamine excretion, which can be used as a good marker of cell activity.

An experiment was carried out to determine the effect of OKG on polyamine levels of traumatised rats. Four groups of rats were used, two were traumatised by fracture of the femur and the other two were controls. One group of traumatised rats and one group of control rats were given a diet supplemented with OKG, while the other two received a normal diet. After six days of feeding, tissues and urine were analysed. It was found that trauma caused a polyamine response seen mainly in muscle tissue, which was paralleled by the amounts excreted in the urine. In the control group, polyamine levels increased when supplemented with OKG, but this was not seen in the trauma groups. Trauma had no significant effects on the polyamine levels of the OKG-fed rats (Table 9.1).

It would seem that OKG was in some way affecting the cellular metabolism of polyamines so that although these levels increased due to trauma; when OKG was given, the increase was absorbed and not measurable.

**Table 9.1** Polyamine (PA) changes seen in traumatised and control rats fed ornithine alpha ketoglutarate (OKG)

| *Group* | *Trauma/control* | *Diet* | *PA changes* |
|---|---|---|---|
| 1 | Trauma | OKG | No change |
| 2 | Trauma | Normal | Increase |
| 3 | Control | OKG | Increase |
| 4 | Control | Normal | No change |

After surgery, trauma or starvation there is a decrease in free glutamine in the peripheral tissues and this has been related to a decrease in protein synthesis in skeletal muscle.[16] Glutamine is supplied continuously to the intestinal mucosa as a respiratory fuel, for cell division, and to protect the intestinal barrier against bacteria.[17] The sharp decrease in muscle glutamine has been related to survival in intensive care patients and it is therefore vital to try to reduce this glutamine decrease after surgery. Thirty-three elective, abdominal surgery patients who were receiving no medication were involved in a study to determine the effects of supplementing post-operative nutrition. The patients were divided into four groups and given total parenteral nutrition (TPN) post-operatively, differing only in the amino acid content. The control group received a commercial amino acid preparation, which contained no glutamine, since it is unstable in solution, a second group received branched chain amino acids, and the two other groups received OKG and glutamine respectively. (Since glutamine is pharmaceutically unstable in solution, for experimental purposes it was acquired as a dry powder vial, which was dissolved in water and added to the amino acid solution immediately before use. OKG however is stable and can be given intravenously in clinical practice.) Immediately before and three days after the operation, a muscle biopsy was taken from above the knee to assess the free glutamine in the knee muscle. In the groups supplied with either glutamine or OKG there was an increase in nitrogen balance and a sparing effect on the glutamine in skeletal muscle, although a significant decrease in glutamine still occurred.

A similar study was carried out with 59 elective abdominal surgery patients,[17] and again a lesser decrease in both glutamine and protein synthesis in skeletal muscle was found in groups receiving TPN supplemented with OKG, alpha ketoglutarate and glutamine. It was suggested that because alpha ketoglutarate is the precursor of glutamine and has the same carbon skeleton, this is the crucial substance for prevention of muscle protein breakdown.

A further study was carried out to see if glutamine and alpha ketoglutarate given post-operatively with a glucose solution, in the absence of TPN would have the same effect.[18] Thirty-three osteoarthritis patients undergoing elective hip replacement entered the study and were given a glucose solution (control) or glucose and glutamine, or glucose and alpha ketoglutarate, post-operatively. Blood samples were taken before and 24 hours after the operation to determine the amino acids in the plasma, and muscle tissue was taken from above the knee to determine the amino acids in skeletal muscle. In the two test groups there was a reduction in the decrease of free glutamine and protein synthesis (measured as a function of ribosome and polyribosome concentration). OKG exerted its actions on protein synthesis even in the absence of TPN.

## Gut functions

Several studies have been carried out to investigate the effects of OKG on gut function and metabolism. Since polyamines are involved in tissue growth, it was thought that feeding with OKG might have an effect on the changes seen in gut function and metabolism, since OKG supplies ornithine, a precursor of polyamines.[19,20] These studies have used the rat as an animal model. In the first study,[19] rats were starved for three days and then fed enterally with a supplement containing either free amino acids or OKG (1 g/kg/day) for seven days. On analysis of the intestinal mucosa, a small but significant increase was noted in the height of the villi. Amino acids were also measured and ornithine and glutamate had increased by over 40% in the OKG-fed rats. There was also a dramatic increase in gamma-aminobutyric acid (GABA). Putrescine was the only polyamine that had a marked increase in concentration.

In the intestinal mucosa, which has no urea cycle, ornithine is metabolised to GABA by two pathways, as shown in Figure 9.3.[19]

To determine the mechanism of action of the OKG, the experiment was repeated, but the animals were fed with OKG plus either aminoguanidine sulfate, which is an inhibitor of the enzyme diamine oxidase (DAO) or 5-fluoromethylornithine (5FMOrn), which blocks ornithine aminotransferase (OAT).

In the presence of aminoguanidine, no GABA was formed and the concentration of putrescine increased, but in the presence of 5FMOrn, GABA was unaffected, although ornithine and putrescine levels increased. This indicated that with OKG the ornithine⇒putrescine⇒GABA

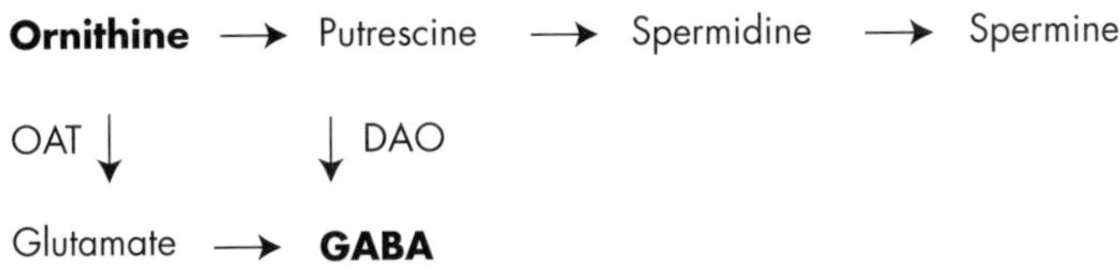


**Figure 9.3** Metabolism of ornithine to gamma aminobutyric acid (GABA). OAT, ornithine aminotransferase; DAO, diamine oxidase.

pathway is preferred, and this probably has a role in the increased mucosal height.

Short bowel syndrome is a malabsorption state resulting from resection of the small intestine. Following surgery, parenteral nutrition is necessary and the remaining bowel compensates for the injury by an increase in mucosa, also called mucosal adaptation, which allows withdrawal of the parenteral feeding.[21] Many structural changes occur in the small intestine after small bowel resection. Since OKG has been shown to exert an effect on the intestinal mucosa, it was thought that it might be useful after this type of surgery. Groups of rats were fed for seven days, after partial resection of the small intestine, followed by starvation for 24 hours. As in the previous experiment, the rats were fed intragastrically with either a diet containing free amino acids or OKG, both diets being isoenergetic, isonitrogenous and containing the same electrolytes and vitamins. After seven days, a section of the terminal ileum was collected for analysis. The OKG diet resulted in increased height of ileal villi (increased mucosal growth) which is dependent on increased putrescine content in the mucosa, as seen in the previous experiment, and was seen to have caused increased early adaptive response to the resection.

In a similar study,[22] OKG was found to offer protection to the intestinal mucosa after vascular occlusion. Intestinal ischaemia leads to loss of protection by the mucosa against bacteria. Before producing intestinal ischaemia by clamping the superior mesenteric artery, either OKG or lysine was fed to male rats. Samples of the intestinal mucosa were removed at the end of the occlusion, and again after 4 hours, and after 24 hours. Increases of spermidine and putrescine were measured immediately after occlusion, increasing even further after 4 hours, before decreasing again. The villi were disconnected and in disarray at the end of occlusion. After only 4 hours, the rats fed with OKG showed restored villi cells, covered with epithelial cells and after 24 hours, although all rats had mucosa that had healed, only the OKG group showed complete restoration. The OKG did not protect the mucosal cells from damage, but did accelerate the repair. The increase in the polyamines measured indicated that these may have been involved in the healing process.

In another study, the effect of OKG on the intestinal barrier was investigated,[23] to see the effect on bacterial translocation, another important factor in intestinal surgery. Sepsis due to the transfer of bacteria is a major cause for concern after small bowel surgery in humans, and can occur due to the failure of the intestinal barrier to provide protection. In this experiment male rats were used for small bowel transplantation. For 24 hours post surgery all animals were fed oral glucose solution. They then received defined formula liquid oral diet (DFD – shown to maintain calorific and protein requirements and weight), standard chow, DFD plus OKG, or standard chow plus OKG. There were six experimental groups of ten rats, all receiving different diets, as shown in Table 9.2.

After two weeks, the animals were killed and the mucosa from the terminal ileum was collected for analysis. Bacterial translocation was measured in each group to determine the effect of oral supplementation on the intestinal barrier. Bacterial translocation was found to be lower in group 6 that received DFD, than in group 5 that received chow, and similar to group 2 that was the chow control group. Whereas intestinal transplantation allows for the optimal amount of bacterial translocation, the addition of OKG to the post-surgery feed significantly reduced these levels. Moreover, the effect was seen to be more marked when the OKG was added to a standard feed rather than DFD.

An investigation was carried out to determine if the advantages of OKG are similar in massive resection of the small bowel.[21] Sixteen rats were used, in which 80% of the small bowel was removed. After 24 hours of receiving water only, enteral feeding began. One group received OKG by continuous flow, and the other received an isonitrogenous diet. After seven days the animals were killed and analysed. The OKG-fed rats showed a significant increase in villi height in the jejunal mucosa and significant improvement in the trophicity of the remaining small bowel, indicating that OKG had accelerated mucosal repair.

Although the studies in the literature have been carried out using animal models, results indicate a possible use for OKG after human intestinal surgery. OKG has a promising role in mucosal adaptation after gut resection and in reducing the time necessary for artificial nutrition. It also appears to improve the nutritional status after surgery and decrease damage to the intestinal barrier, while improving healing.

**Table 9.2** Groups and feeds of the experimental rats[23]

| *Group* | *Procedure* | *Feed* |
|---|---|---|
| Group 1 | Non-transplanted | DFD |
| Group 2 | Non-transplanted | Chow |
| Group 3 | Transplanted | DFD |
| Group 4 | Transplanted | Chow |
| Group 5 | Transplanted | DFD + OKG |
| Group 6 | Transplanted | Chow + OKG |

OKG, ornithine alpha ketoglutarate; DFD, defined formula liquid oral diet.

## Cancer

Patients with cancer often experience a loss of lean body mass of as much as 75% of their previous (healthy) body mass, which may be related to a decreased food intake, or substrate consumption by the tumour, and is different in different tumours. This leads to decreased tolerance to treatments such as radiation, surgery or chemotherapy as well as increased morbidity. Since OKG has been shown to improve nitrogen balance in other catabolic states, such as trauma, it was thought that it might have a place in the nutritional support of cancer patients. Two rat experiments with OKG have been published,[24,25] which provide a preliminary indication that there may be a role for OKG supplementation in cancer patients. In the first study, OKG had no effect on the tumour growth but showed a decrease in muscle protein breakdown. In the second, one group of rats had the tumours surgically removed and OKG supplementation improved nitrogen balance in this group, but not in the group that did not undergo surgery.

## Growth

OKG enhances protein synthesis and nitrogen balance, and ornithine is involved in polyamine synthesis, which is related to the regulation of cell growth and tissue protein synthesis. It follows, therefore, that OKG may have a role in growth patterns. An animal model was used in which 16 growing rats were fed freely for seven days.[26] Half received a liquid oral diet and the others were fed an isonitrogenous diet, in which the nitrogen was replaced by OKG. Results showed that in the OKG group there was a 16% increase in food intake and an 11% increase in nitrogen retention. From the fourth day of OKG supplementation, the OKG group grew better, showing an overall 15% weight gain over the week. The urinary polyamines, putrescine and spermidine, were also increased, indicating a rise in cellular activity. Supplemented rats showed unchanged plasma ornithine levels, however, indicating its efficient metabolism.

Unexplained growth disturbances often occur in children receiving TPN. A small study was carried out[27,28] in which five boys and a girl were given supplemented TPN, to see its effect on growth. The children were all pre-pubertal and were aged between 9 and 16 years. They had all been on home TPN for between five and ten years, for impaired intestinal absorption resulting from Crohn's disease or short bowel syndrome. For at least one year before the start of the study, all children showed decreased linear growth. During the first five months of the study, the children were given a supplement of 15 g/day OKG. Compatibility and stability tests indicated no problems for the pharmacist to add the OKG to the home TPN bags prior to the weekly home delivery. For the second five months, the TPN remained the same, except for the OKG.

All but one child increased in height in part one of the study. (The child who did not subsequently died from liver cirrhosis and should not have been included in the study due to his abnormal liver function.) Two children continued to grow even when the supplementation was stopped. Weight increase was noted in both parts of the study. There were no side-effects from the OKG and it was well tolerated by all children. None of the children were malnourished and they all showed the appropriate height/weight ratios and skinfold thickness. Testosterone and estradiol levels were the same before and after the test period, indicating that height increase was not due to puberty growth spurts. However the two children who continued to grow in the second half of the study may have been about to start puberty. It was suggested that OKG acts on the insulin-like growth factor (IGF-1), which is related to an increase in growth rate. For more conclusive results a much larger trial is required in which puberty effects can be ruled out.

### Immune response

As already discussed, glutamine is depleted in injury states. In these situations there is an efflux of glutamine from the muscle to meet the extra requirements of the other organs. Since glutamine is also necessary for providing energy in immune cells and fibroblasts, when the levels decrease dramatically there may be inhibition of immune function. There may therefore be a use for OKG to provide additional glutamine supplies in sepsis and infection. To test this hypothesis 12 rats were infected with an injection of *Escherichia coli* endotoxin.[29] A control group received saline and remained uninfected. After a day of fasting, by which time the infected rats showed clinical signs of infection, such as diarrhoea and decreased activity, enteral feeding was started. The infected group was further divided into two; one received a supplement of OKG (0.5 g/kg/day) and the other received glycine. After 48 hours the rats were killed, and blood was collected from the neck for analysis. Muscle, thymus, liver and small intestine were removed. Results showed that in the infected rats fed glycine, there was a 30% decrease in thymus weight, which corresponded to a marked reduction of immune function.

In the group fed OKG, this decrease was not seen. Also in the infected rats, the liver weight was unchanged but the intestinal weight increased. Muscle amino acids showed a marked decrease in the infected rats not fed OKG, with glutamine being depleted by 30% and arginine by 56%. OKG supplementation restored these amounts, to concentrations higher than those seen in the control rats. There was no difference noted in the concentrations of glutamate, proline and ornithine in the muscle, or of glutamate, glutamine and arginine in the plasma. The reason for this may be the very low dose of OKG used.

There seems to be a correlation between thymus weight and arginine and glutamine concentration. Since OKG is a precursor of these two amino acids, these experiments suggest a possible role for OKG in septic states to prevent thymus involution and improve immune function.

## Conclusions

It has been shown that OKG is a very promising nutritional supplement that has been used with success in many different experimental and clinical situations. The only side-effect noted is diarrhoea, in doses above 15 g/day.[5] By providing physiological metabolites, OKG has a role in trauma and surgical patients, as well as in wound healing, malnutrition and growth, and even possibly in cancer patients. The results from experiments showing the effect of OKG supplementation on the intestinal tract are impressive. Research in this area continues and OKG will perhaps one day be included in standard feeds for hospitalised and chronically ill patients.

However, those promoting this nutraceutical as a sports supplement do so with no evidence for their declarations, and instead base claims on the medical evidence of the use of OKG to prevent protein breakdown and improve nutritional status, as well as to improve recovery time from injury and illness.

## References

1. Cyberpump. The HIT FAQ. http://cyberpump.com/hitfaq/ (accessed 1 September 2001).
2. Le Boucher J, Cynober L. Ornithine α-ketoglutarate: the puzzle. *Nutrition* 1998; 14: 870–873.
3. Cynober L A, Ornithine α-ketoglutarate. In: Cynober L A, ed. *Amino Acid Metabolism and Therapy in Health and Nutritional Disease*. Boca Raton: CRC Press, 1995: 385–398.

4. De Bandt J P, Coudray-Lucas C, Lioret N, *et al.* A randomized controlled trial of the influence of the mode of enteral ornithine α-ketoglutarate administration in burn patients. *J Nutr* 1998; 128: 563–569.
5. Cynober L. Ornithine α-ketoglutarate in nutritional support. *Nutrition* 1991; 7: 313–322.
6. Wernerman J. Alpha ketoglutarate in the treatment of post-operative and critically ill patients. *Clin Nutr* 1993; 12: 58–59.
7. Cynober L, Coudray-Lucas C, de Bandt J P, *et al.* Action of ornithine α-ketoglutarate, ornithine hydrochloride, and calcium α-ketoglutarate on plasma amino acid and hormonal patterns in healthy subjects. *J Am Coll Nutr* 1990; 9: 2–12.
8. Jeevanandam M, Holaday N J, Petersen S R. Ornithine-α-ketoglutarate (OKG) supplementation is more effective than its component salts in traumatized rats. *J Nutr* 1996; 126: 2141–2150.
9. Cynober L. The use of α-ketoglutarate salts in clinical; nutrition and metabolic care. *Clin Nutr Metab Care* 1999; 2: 33–37.
10. Cynober L. Amino acid metabolism in thermal burns. *J Parenteral Enteral Nutr* 1989; 13: 196–205.
11. Cynober L, Saizy R, Dinh F N, *et al.* Effect of enterally administered ornithine α-ketoglutarate on plasma and urinary amino acid levels after burn injury. *J Trauma* 1984; 24: 590–596.
12. Cynober L, Lioret N, Coudray Lucas C, *et al.* Action of ornithine α-ketoglutarate on protein metabolism in burn patients. *Nutrition* 1987; 3: 187–191.
13. Donati L, Zeigler F, Pongelli G, *et al.* Nutritional and clinical efficacy of ornithine alpha-ketoglutarate in severe burn patients. *Clin Nutr* 1999; 18: 307–311.
14. Le Bricon T, Coudray-Lucas C, Lioret N, *et al.* Ornithine α-ketoglutarate metabolism after enteral administration in burn patients: bolus compared with continuous infusion. *Am J Clin Nutr* 1997; 65: 512–518.
15. Jeevanandam M, Holaday N J, Ali M R. Altered tissue polyamine levels due to ornithine α-ketoglutarate in traumatised growing rats. *Metab Clin Exp* 1992; 41: 1204–1209.
16. Wernerman J, Hammarkvist F, Ali M R, *et al.* Glutamine and ornithine α-ketoglutarate but not branched chain amino acids reduce the loss of muscle glutamine after surgical trauma. *Metabolism* 1989; 38: 63–66.
17. Wernerman J, Hammarkvist F, Vinnars E. Alpha ketoglutarate and post-operative muscle catabolism. *Lancet* 1990; 335: 701–703.
18. Blomqvist B I, Hammarqvist F, von der Decken A, *et al.* Glutamine and α-ketoglutarate prevent the decrease in muscle free glutamine concentration and influence protein synthesis after total hip replacement. *Metabolism* 1995; 44: 1215–1222.
19. Raul F, Gosse F, Galluser M, *et al.* Functional and metabolic changes in intestinal mucosa of rats after enteral administration of ornithine α-ketoglutarate salt. *J Parenteral Enteral Nutr* 1995; 19: 145–150.
20. Czernichow B, Nsi-Emvo E, Galluser M, *et al.* Enteral supplementation with ornithine α-ketoglutarate improves the early adaptive response to resection. *Gut* 1997; 40: 67–72.
21. Dumas F, de Bandt J P, Colomb V, *et al.* Enteral ornithine α-ketoglutarate

enhances intestinal adaptation to massive resection in rats. *Metab Clin Exp* 1998; 47: 1366–1371.
22. Duranton B, Schleiffer R, Gosse F, *et al.* Preventative administration of ornithine α-ketoglutarate improves intestinal mucosal repair after transient ischemia in rats. *Crit Care Med* 1998; 26: 120–125.
23. De Oca J, Bettonica C, Cuadrado S, *et al.* Effect of oral supplementation of ornithine α-ketoglutarate on the intestinal barrier after orthotopic small bowel transplantation. *Transplantation* 1997; 63: 636–639.
24. Le Bricon T, Cynober L, Baracos V E. Ornithine α-ketoglutarate limits muscle protein breakdown without stimulating tumour growth in rats bearing *Yoshida* ascites hepatoma. *Metabolism* 1994; 43: 899–905.
25. Le Bricon T, Cynober L, Field C J, *et al.* Supplemental nutrition with ornithine α-ketoglutarate in rats with cancer-associated cachexia: surgical treatment of the tumour improves efficacy of nutritional support. *J Nutr* 1995; 125: 2999–3010.
26. Jeevanandam M, Ali M R, Ramias L, *et al.* Efficacy of ornithine α-ketoglutarate as a dietary supplement in growing rats. *Clin Nutr* 1991; 10: 155–161.
27. Moukarzel A, Goulet O, Cynober L, *et al.* Positive effects of ornithine α-ketoglutarate in paediatric patients on parenteral nutrition with failure to thrive. *Clin Nutr* 1993; 12: 59–60.
28. Moukarzel A, Goulet O, Salas J S, *et al.* Growth retardation in children receiving long-term parenteral nutrition: effects of ornithine α-ketoglutarate. *Am J Clin Nutr* 1994; 60: 408–413.
29. Lasnier E, Coudray Lucas C, le Boucher J, *et al.* Ornithine α-ketoglutarate counteracts thymus involution and glutamine depletion in endotoxemic rats. *Clin Nutr* 1996; 15: 197–200.

# 10

# Conclusions

Although a few of the nutraceuticals being promoted for their health aspects have been reviewed, many more are also available and the amount of literature published in this field grows daily.

Speculation on who the winners of the nutraceutical venture will be is becoming a popular topic in newspapers discussing the pharmaceutical industry. Because new medicines are harder to find and more expensive and riskier to develop than ever before, many companies which have produced conventional pharmaceuticals in the past are now merging to survive or are turning to nutraceuticals, for example Du Pont, Abbott Laboratories and Warner Lambert.[1] Novartis Consumer Health, the nutrition division of the Swiss drugs group Novartis, announced a joint venture with the Quaker Oats Company in February 2000, forming the Altus Food Company to sell functional foods in the United States. This venture was the first union between a drugs company and a food company. Novartis Consumer Health has also launched the Aviva range of functional foods that are available in supermarkets and pharmacies. Mergers of this kind offer the companies involved a very large market and more alliances of this kind are likely, as joint ventures help to share knowledge, risk, flexibility, expertise and cost.[2]

Datamonitor, a website that follows market trends, estimates the nutraceutical market at $17 billion and Dr De Felice of the Foundation for Innovation in Medicine (see Chapter 1), speaking at a conference in 1998 put the figure at $250 billion in America alone.[3]

In the UK, the functional food market was estimated to be worth £255 million at the end of 1999, based on foods to which ingredients have been added for a specific health benefit, and foods that have been modified or processed for a health benefit.[2] Other sources report that sales of food supplements in 2000 showed a reduction of 1.5% (possibly due to scares about high doses of certain nutrients and warning of interactions with herbal medicines), but the market was still very large and estimated at a value of £305.3 million.[4]

Although these estimates vary widely, the nutraceutical market is undoubtedly very large and growing. As companies increase in size more jobs may be created, but the real impact of nutraceuticals on pharmacy will be in the community. If restrictions on health claims were lifted, the market could be flooded with products that have no evidence for their claims. This is very unlikely, but rather it has been suggested that a move from dietary supplements, sold in health-food shops and most pharmacies, to nutraceuticals aimed at the prescription market could occur. This would not necessarily be in the manufacturers' best interest, as it would limit the size of the market. However, many indications under research are for serious disease states for which self-medication is inappropriate. Examples include flaxseed oil and carnitine for cardiovascular disease, ornithine alpha ketoglutarate for post surgery and antioxidants for the prevention of cancer. At present, consumers may try dietary supplements for many indications believing them to be safer than synthetic substances and this presumption of safety is erroneous. Consumer-friendly terms must be used to relay scientifically correct, proven information. Government support is required for increased research in these areas and in the long term, reduced health costs would justify the money spent.

Some of these supplements are also available as functional foods, which are foods that have been altered in some way to increase health.[2] One example is Columbus Healthier eggs, introduced in October 1998 by Dean Farms, a privately owned company in Tring, Hertfordshire, UK. These eggs are rich in ω3 fatty acids as a result of the hens being fed a diet rich in ω3 fats. All major British supermarkets now stock these eggs. Similarly, OmegaTech has launched DHA Gold eggs, rich in both ω3 fatty acids and docosahexaenoic acid. Another example was the introduction of Burgen bread in September 1997 by Allied Bakeries, the largest bread manufacturer in the UK. This bread is a wholegrain loaf with soya and flaxseed, which was very successful commercially in Australia. The pack claims 'high in natural plant oestrogens, believed to help menopausal symptoms'.

In spite of repeated public health messages to increase the amount of fruits and vegetables in the diet, consumption does not seem to have changed and is particularly low amongst high-risk cancer patients and adolescents. Moreover, since increasing fruit and vegetable intake tends to be difficult for some people, supplements could be a way to provide many of the benefits provided by the fruits and vegetables themselves.[5]

In either case, whether prescribed by a doctor or self-selected, the challenge is to be up to date with research developments so that both conventional practitioners as well as members of the public are able to receive accurate information.

## References


1. Brower B. Nutraceuticals: poised for a healthy slice of the market. *Nature Biotechnol* 1998; 16: 728–733.
2. *Mintel Market Intelligence*, Functional Foods, March 2000: 1–47.
3. Mannion M. Nutraceutical revolution continues at Foundation for Innovation in Medicine Conference. *Am J Nat Med* 1998; 5: 30–33.
4. Anon. OTC sales growth matches inflation. *Pharm J* 2001; 266: 571.
5. Inserra P F, Jiang S, Solkoff D, *et al*. Immune function in elderly smokers and nonsmokers improves during supplementation with fruit and vegetable extracts. *Integrative Med* 1999; 2: 3–10.

# Index